JO AND ALICE KINGSLEY

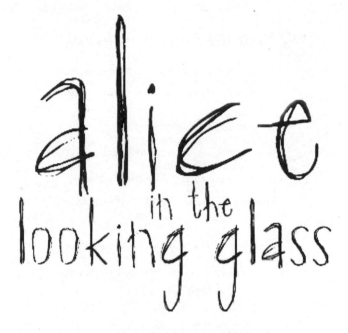

alice
in the
looking glass

A MOTHER AND
DAUGHTER'S EXPERIENCE
OF ANOREXIA

PIATKUS

For Jean

Copyright © 2005 by Jo and Alice Kingsley

First published in Great Britain in 2005 by
Piatkus Books Ltd
5 Windmill Street, London W1T 2JA
email: info@piatkus.co.uk

The moral right of the author has been asserted

A catalogue record for this book is available from the British Library

ISBN 0 7499 2637 6 HB
ISBN 0 7499 2682 1 PB

Text design by Goldust Design

This book has been printed on paper manufactured
with respect for the environment using wood from
managed sustainable resources

Typeset by Phoenix Photosetting, Chatham, Kent
Printed and bound in Great Britain by
Biddles Ltd, King's Lynn, Norfork

CONTENTS

'Experience is a hard teacher because she gives
the test first, the lesson afterwards.'

VERNON LAW

ACKNOWLEDGEMENTS

With tremendous thanks to the team of health professionals at the unit for their patience, understanding and consistency. Thanks to Beth, Jenny, Ian and all our friends, without whom this book would have no end. And finally our thanks to Gill Bailey and Jo Brooks at Piatkus, and to our copy editor Jan Cutler, for making this all possible.

Extract from *Anorexia Nervosa: A Survival Guide for Families, Friends and Sufferers* (Psychology Press, 1977, repr. Brunner-Routledge, 2003) reproduced by kind permission of Janet Treasure and Psychology Press.

PART ONE
A Mother's Experience

Introduction

It has been important for me to write down Alice's and my story before I forgot the trials and tribulations we have experienced during her illness and what we hope will be her recovery. Throughout the anorexic journey that we have shared together there have been long periods of huge despair, guilt, anger and, for me as a mother of a much-loved child, sheer terror. It had never been my intention to write a book about our experiences but, during the five long years of Alice's illness between the ages of 14 and 19, I have read many books about the condition, and the more information I gathered, the more I came to appreciate that there was no guaranteed solution to achieve recovery. Nevertheless, I did find some valuable pointers.

I began by writing notes in diary form, recounting the turbulent and completely bewildering world I experienced when Alice was aged between 11 and 17. Although she knew that I had written this account, at the time she had no desire to read it for herself and there was no opportunity to ask how different her interpretation might have been from mine. I hoped that perhaps in time we might discuss what I had written but I never expected that Alice would put her own analysis down on paper. However, this was the

3

approach she wanted to take and once she had begun there was no stopping her.

Our accounts have resulted in two very different pictures of obsessive-compulsive disorder and anorexia nervosa. Although Alice and I have written our accounts for different reasons and from different angles, there is no escaping the enormity of dependence we have put on the professionals. Hindsight is a wonderful thing; we can now appreciate the exceptional expertise and care they provided, though at the time it was not always so obvious. I hope that between us we have reflected the significance of the professionals' role.

I am not a professional or a 'carer'; I am simply a mum who loves her children and who found herself in completely unknown territory. Obsessive-compulsive disorder and anorexia nervosa were illnesses that I had never previously encountered or experienced in any shape or form, but both of them came to call on Alice. I wish to pass on my experiences as a mother of a child suffering from these illnesses, and to share all my doubts, failures and anxieties as well as the successes, in the hope that I might offer support to other families who are going through the same trauma.

The first major hurdle was trying to find out what on earth was going wrong with Alice. Obsessive-compulsive disorder (OCD) was easy to diagnose once we accepted that we needed professional help – Alice was 11 years old. Anorexia nervosa, however, was far more furtive in its appearance; although I was convinced that something was terribly wrong way before the illness had taken a grip, I was at a loss as to what the problem was. By the time we had found the professional help required, Alice was desperately ill and approaching 15. I began to read whatever I could find that seemed relevant, and I quickly became immersed in statistics, what my role should be as a mother of an adolescent anorexic child and, finally, the information that I feared the most: possible explanations for a child becoming anorexic. The statistics made terrifying reading: 1-2 per cent of the population suffer from anorexia nervosa; after five years, on average more than 40 per cent of anorexics will have recovered, 30 per cent will remain quite severely affected by their illness and 20 per cent will still be underweight and without their periods. There is a 10 per cent mortality rate, which represents incidents of suicide as well as complications caused by the starvation that is the hallmark of their illness. Where was Alice going to fit into these statistics? I learnt that early diagnosis was an advantage in treating the illness, but I knew that it had taken almost a year to find the professional expertise we needed. Hidden among the facts and figures was perhaps the hardest part: accepting that Alice suffered from a 'mental illness'.

In my search for understanding, particular words often appeared in books that I read. My interpretation of the primary role of a parent caring for a child suffering from anorexia was 'support', but what did that mean? I had always supported the children but this was new territory; was I meant to be a prop, a disciplinarian or simply to encourage as I always had before? 'Normality' was another word that often cropped up and drove me to distraction. How was it possible to find any normality when everything that I had taken for granted as normal had disappeared?

And finally – I came to the possible causes for anorexia nervosa. We didn't fit every category; we had no previous history of anorexia in our family, Alice had not been abused or bullied to my knowledge, I don't think she even suffered from low self-esteem; and the 'perfectionist' trait had never been apparent before the arrival of OCD. However, we did fit into the 'dysfunctional family' syndrome: I was divorced and had a partner. In none of the books I had read could I find the answers to my questions: was anybody else finding this as excruciatingly difficult to manage as me? Was I doing everything wrong? Why wasn't Alice improving like some of her fellow patients?

In my story that follows I have described the difficulties I encountered while attempting to encompass the complexities of Alice's condition and the overriding memory of loneliness and isolation I felt during my search.

CHAPTER 1
All's Not Well

Born in 1954, I enjoyed an idyllic childhood living with my American mother, English father and older sister in Newcastle upon Tyne. I married David when I was 24; we met when I was working for auction houses and fine art specialists – work that I didn't particularly enjoy and didn't really feel suited me. He was great company and I had absolutely no doubt that between us we would make a happy and successful combination. Our first daughter, Beth, was born the following year, and I realised that I had now found my niche – I loved being married and a mother. Jenny arrived the following year. David's career meant that as a family we moved around the country, and we were successful and upwardly mobile – a happy family.

On 29 May 1986 Alice was born. I remember thinking at the time of her birth that my life was now complete; I had everything I could possibly want. But I was wrong. When Alice was only nine months old my husband left home, leaving his work telephone number but otherwise no other point of contact. I was devastated. I wonder now whether Alice heard the worst of my thoughts: because she was only a small baby I could tell her the truth and not the story I had given Beth and Jenny, who believed their father was away on a business trip. I remember cutting the grass in our large garden with Alice in a baby carrier on my back while I complained bitterly about her father deserting us for a 19-year-old secretary who wore hot-pants. I kept the news from my mother for the first few months after David had left because she was caring for my father, who was suffering with Parkinson's disease, and I felt that she had more than enough problems of her own to cope with. So I bore my problems alone.

David visited the children occasionally and, after about six months, just as I was beginning to take control of my life again, he came home. Three months later, my father died and although we attempted to rebuild our relationship, after six years it was apparent that our marriage had failed. David was as unhappy as I was when I asked him for a divorce. Beth was 13, Jenny 12 and Alice 7 when he finally left. We had a horse, two ponies, our dog Basil and not a lot of money.

David quickly remarried and left us very much to our own devices. He and I rarely spoke, and any conversations we did have were antagonistic. We rowed over everything: a 'wish you were here' postcard that the children received after his marriage, to which they were not invited, infuriated me. I was also incensed when Alice returned home with a gerbil the first time she stayed with David and her new step-mother. She was thrilled, but I loathed anything resembling rats – surely her father knew me well enough to know that! Nevertheless, despite my bitterness, I hope that I always portrayed to the children that their father had always loved them, even though our marriage had failed. My foremost aim was to keep their day-to-day lives as close as possible to how they had been before.

The girls and I moved to a small house, with a field for the horses, which I couldn't really afford but which gave the children a great deal of pleasure. I had various jobs between school hours, varying from apple picking to cataloguing for a local book dealer, but I was very aware that I needed to find a career that could support us financially and this was a constant worry for me.

During this time I began to work for Ian, a farmer, as a farm secretary, adjusting the hours to fit around the school days and holidays. Like me, his marriage had broken up. He was easy-going, kind, uncomplicated and with a permanent smile on his face; we shared our anxieties, and I liked him. He was there on every difficult day I experienced: divorce day, moving day and all the other days in between. His visits became more and more frequent and it wasn't long before the children guessed that we were no longer 'just friends'. Life was surprisingly uncomplicated, the children were showing no obvious signs of trauma from the divorce and I was happier than I had been for a long time.

When a house in the middle of Ian's farm came up for sale, the children were enthusiastic as, although it was in a more isolated position than our current village home, it had better paddocks and stabling for the horses. I couldn't quite afford the asking price, so Ian offered to make up the difference.

It was perfect; I would also be closer to Ian, who by then was divorced and living with two of his children, Olivia, aged 17 and Luke, aged 14. I felt very lucky to have three wonderful children, a relationship with someone I loved and respected, and enough regular income to keep us secure.

And so we moved to Chittering Farm. It is still our home, and we all love it, but the past nine years have seen a gradual change, perhaps most simply noticed in the way I now sort out the socks, mentally saying, 'Alice, Jenny and Beth' whereas nine years ago it was 'Beth, Jenny and Alice'. Ian is still waiting for me to sort his socks. I hope that Beth, Jenny, Ian and his family will understand that I am now going to continue my story from the perspective of Alice and myself. It is an easy sentence to write but it is presuming an enormous amount because they have contributed so much and in so many ways. Without their combined support, the struggle would have seemed insurmountable on many occasions and the consequences have severely disrupted their own individual expectations and aspirations.

Before I ever met Alice she had worried me. I had suffered a couple of miscarriages before her birth and I thought Alice had gone the same way. When I was 12 weeks pregnant I had my third miscarriage. It was the same procedure as before: the bleeding and pain, a trip to the hospital, a D&C and home again with a desperate feeling of emptiness and loss. Except this time I couldn't quite understand why about eight weeks later I felt so hungry. I didn't feel I was eating more than usual but my waistband continued to get tighter.

Eventually I decided to visit the GP and ask whether there was any chance that I could still be pregnant. It was an amusing conversation and I was told it was just a problem with my hormones settling down. Except that my hormones just wouldn't settle down, and, after another visit, the GP suggested that perhaps I should have a scan just to give me some peace of mind. The scan showed that I was 22 weeks pregnant. The consultant explained that I had actually been pregnant with twins and had miscarried one of them. He was irritated when he noticed a packet of cigarettes in my bag. I stopped smoking immediately and prayed that the baby had survived a clinical procedure that should have removed any trace of his or her existence. It made for a very long and worrying pregnancy.

There had been no problems with Beth's or Jenny's birth. When I went into labour with Alice, however, I was rushed into hospital, as her heartbeat was unsatisfactory and I needed to be induced. I was convinced that my child would be badly scarred or damaged, and I could not find the confidence to produce the baby on my own, so I asked for an epidural. I gave birth to a beautiful baby girl; she was perfect except for the tiniest fault with her baby toe.

My new arrival peered at me from her cot with one eye open and one eye shut – and screamed. I longed to hold her but was experiencing more pain than I had ever known. It seemed an eternity before anyone realised that I was haemorrhaging, and all I can remember is panic, blood and being hurried off to theatre. For both of us the pregnancy and delivery were immensely stressful.

We called our third daughter Alice because we were reminded of *Alice in Wonderland* – she was indeed something wonderful: a miracle.

As a baby Alice cried quite a lot and preferred to be with me rather than passed around for others to hold. However, by the ripe old age of two years Alice had found her feet; she was the most uncomplicated, amusing toddler to have about the place. Her greatest little friend was Nuala – the daughter of a great friend of mine and three months older than Alice – and the two of them played in their own imaginary world for hours. They didn't really like toys, but they loved chatting, sometimes in dens and tree houses in the garden, and usually with an American accent. As Alice grew up she became a tremendous mimic and often had us in stitches with her antics. It is so difficult to describe the characteristics of a child, but maybe Alice's are best summarised by a light-hearted conversation the four of us had when Alice was about eight or nine. We discussed whether we thought any of us had been in this world before, and we agreed that probably out of the four of us I had made the fewest visits: I seemed to get myself into muddles and obviously was something of an amateur; Beth came next, as she was slightly better at managing life but would benefit from a couple more practice runs; Jenny we thought had probably been here quite a few times – she was a capable soul; but there was absolutely no question among the four of us that Alice was the old timer: she had life sorted.

Alice was ten when we moved to the farm, and the first year passed uneventfully. Beth was studying for A levels and had the advantage of a boyfriend with a car. Jenny was busy with GCSEs and the main love of her life – the ponies. When we moved I asked Alice whether she wanted to stay at her old primary school or transfer to a new one for her last year. It had come as no surprise when she decided to try the new school. 'I've always wondered what it would be like to be a "new girl",' she said, and off she went. She expanded her already comprehensive network of friends, and her main problem was keeping up with her busy social life.

The following year, Alice began secondary school. Apart from a little disappointment that neither of her sisters would be there because the school did not offer sixth-form facilities, she was excited and pleased that she would have the friends from both her primary schools under the same roof. I had no worries when she went off in her new uniform for her first day at school. Beth and Jenny had been very happy there and I was sure Alice would follow the same route.

During her first term Alice, then aged 11, started to develop her rituals or 'rigmaroles', as they were to become known in our family. They began with her having difficulty walking in and out of doors from one room to another, and she would have to repeat the process four times, changing steps each time to get into the room; she would also turn the light switch on and off four times, and check the phone four times. After about a month it was obvious that they were becoming a problem, and Alice was also certainly much less social than her usual self. I didn't know about OCD at this stage and the whole process was completely baffling to me. Her schoolwork and homework became totally muddled, with endless crossings-out and, although she spent hours working on it, the teachers began to comment on the deterioration in her work. One morning, after I'd taken my older daughters to the school bus stop, I returned home to find Alice sitting on her bed battling to do up her shirt buttons and school tie; she was extremely upset and I knew that the time had come to see the GP.

The doctor was helpful and reassuring. She explained that these rituals were quite common among children and teenagers and so long as Alice managed to control the rituals, and not the other way round, she would probably come out of it. If she lost the battle, the GP suggested seeing a psychiatrist. Over a period of six months the rigmaroles gradually did begin to disappear, and Alice returned to her more normal self. I don't know how she managed to control them but I suspect she had the strength of mind to overcome them, and she certainly did not want to go and see a 'shrink'. At the time, I put the whole experience down to just one of those things that happen, although a great friend did warn me to keep a close look-out for further problems.

The next two years saw a change at home. Ian was often stressed and disclosed that he had suffered from a nervous breakdown 15 years ago, when he suffered from panic attacks. I realised that he was a very different man from my husband, who had been largely self-sufficient: Ian needed to talk problems through with me and be with me. More of my time was taken up with the farm. Ian worked extraordinarily hard and he liked us both to spend Saturdays going to rugby matches. As a result, there was less time for the children and their activities. Most evenings Ian and Luke came for supper; sometimes we saw Olivia, which was always a bonus, but she had begun university and was away. Those evenings were often strained because we didn't share the same interests and it was difficult for us all to mix and have fun.

A completely unexpected trip to the States brought the rather tense atmosphere to a head. I received an invitation from my godmother asking us to visit her in Boston and meet her family in San Francisco. My mother had often spoken fondly of her days before she married my father and came to live in England, and I was thrilled that I was going to have the opportunity to see her heritage. Beth, Jenny and Alice could not contain their excitement; holidays had never really featured and the prospect of a two-week trip to the States was beyond their wildest expectations. Unfortunately, Ian did not share our enthusiasm; he was angry that he had not been invited and thought we should not accept my godmother's offer. We will differ to this day as to who was right and who was wrong; he will never forgive my decision to go but I felt that it was too wonderful an opportunity for us to miss, and so we went.

Ian telephoned every day but it was not until we met at Heathrow on our return that it became obvious that he had really suffered during our absence. He looked dreadful and I realised that I had pushed his boundaries of coping to the limit; he had really missed me. There was no question of a jolly evening with the four of us sharing our adventure with Ian; it was as if we had never been. However, he was so relieved to see me and I was appalled that the holiday had caused him such misery. Within three days of our return we decided to get married and put the past behind us. We shared our exciting news with all the children and received a somewhat mixed response, but no slamming of doors.

Plans were drawn up to extend Chittering Farm. We needed to provide accommodation for six children (Ian hoped that his youngest daughter Heidi, who lived with her mother nearby, would stay with us from time to time). Before long we were involved with builders and diggers. I suppose my children rather wished their house could stay the same as it was, and Ian's children didn't really want to move, so the project was met bleakly from both sides. As old walls came down and new ones went up, the tension increased. Ian and Luke spent hours tapping walls and scrutinising developments. Although Beth largely escaped the invasion because she had begun university, Jenny was having a bad time: she had grown too big for her pony so it had to be sold, and as Ian regularly pointed out, I really couldn't afford the upkeep of three ponies. She had set her sights on becoming a vet so needed excellent A level grades. Tolerance was never her strongest point and she found the combination of builders all day and Ian and Luke discussing farming and building every night irritating, so she decided to remove herself from the evening conversations. Alice plodded on, making cups of tea for the builders when she got home from school – the cups were usually half-empty by the time she had struggled through the scaffolding to deliver them. She, too, decided to opt out of the evening-meal saga and decided to have her supper watching television on her own. I tried desperately hard to change the atmosphere that we were creating. I spoke to the girls and to Ian, pointing out that we all had to make a special effort to include everyone in our conversations, but I completely failed at bridging the gap between the two families. I dreaded the prospect of a home life filled yet again with animosity, and so, regrettably, I asked Ian to postpone the wedding until the negative waves had settled a little. It was a cruel request; Ian had paid for the extension and wanted the security of a home and a wife who loved him. All I wanted was a content and secure home for everyone.

By now Alice was 13 and there had been no signs of any recurrence of her OCD. She was happily settled into school life and participated in any extra sporting activities she could. She had decided not to pursue the competitive aspect of riding, which had taken up so much of her sisters' spare time. Her opinion was that she had spent enough wet weekends watching Beth and Jenny jump over fences. We still had Beth's horse and one small Welsh mountain pony and, though Alice didn't ride a great deal, she was more than happy to do her share of mucking out. The aggression at home had subsided and to an extent I think we were all getting along better. Ian's fiftieth birthday was approaching, which filled him with doom, so he decided that as we hadn't had a wedding he would throw a big birthday party instead.

The evening of 14 September 2000 is the last night we can all remember when everyone was well and, given the circumstances, happy. We decorated the barn, Ian's friends reunited to form a rock band from his younger days, and all the children and their various girl- and boyfriends did whatever they could to help provide a memorable evening. Although Alice didn't have a boyfriend, she participated to the full. She looked rather like a young antelope ready to spring; it was obvious that she was going to be tall and leggy. It was a wonderful evening, Ian smiled and we were all delighted that at least he had celebrated something.

The long demise began with the sudden departure of Basil our dear old loyal dog at the end of October. Perhaps he knew what lay ahead and decided to make a timely exit. The house seemed quieter than ever, Jenny had left for university in London the month before – disappointed because her veterinary applications had not been successful, and about to embark on a degree in biochemistry instead. Ian was on his own at home, too, because Luke had begun his degree in agriculture. Alice had been dreading the prospect of being the only one left behind and I knew it was important that she mustn't feel excluded at home.

However, Alice, now 14, decided to plot her own course. This time it didn't take the form of rigmaroles; it was more of a continued gradual quiet withdrawal. I knew all was not right, but I couldn't pinpoint the problem. I shared my concerns with Ian but his view was that she was a typical 14-year-old who was being rather difficult and looking for attention. It was difficult to argue against his opinion and I hoped that her withdrawal was just a passing spell.

In November Alice's changing personality made its first real appearance. Most unusually, the three of us (Ian, myself and Alice) had arranged to go to the London Eye with good friends and their son. What should have been a super day turned out to be a disaster. I was totally bemused by Alice's behaviour: she was quiet, grumpy and obviously not enjoying herself at all, and I remember saying when we went out for supper that night that I wondered why Alice was spending so long in the ladies.

We went to Newcastle to visit my mother and my sister's family for Christmas and by then Alice was already looking thinner. The visit had always been anticipated with excitement in the past, but Alice was not her usual bubbly self; she was tremendously helpful with the Christmas preparations, very polite, but so quiet. The girls planned to visit their father over New Year but Alice was most reluctant to go. She hated the prospect of another long car drive and she looked tired. However, she was persuaded to join her sisters, who pointed out that they had not seen their dad for nearly a year and they really should all go. I rarely communicated with their father, but on this occasion I decided to write him a letter explaining that I was worried about Alice and asking him to keep a close eye on her.

Very gradually Alice was removing more and more from her diet. Without my really noticing, she asked me to spread the Flora more thinly, then sandwich fillings began to disappear, and then crisps and snacks were left out. I was happy to meet her wishes. I knew that her sisters had said in passing 'Don't put the pounds on now, Alice – so much harder to lose later on!' and I hoped that it might improve her state of mind, though she had only ever been an average size, and had never been overweight.

Although the lunches grew smaller, Alice still ate a large supper and the possibility of an eating disorder never once crossed my mind. A 'stylish' image was not particularly important to us as a family, as we preferred to spend money on the horses rather than typical fashion accessories. Alice was not particularly fashion conscious or influenced by fashionable body shapes and sizes as far as I was aware.

Alice's school was organising a ski trip for the following spring. It was something she had always wanted to do and I hoped that booking her a place would improve her mood and give her something to look forward to. I wondered if perhaps something was going wrong at school which Alice wasn't prepared to tell me, but when I asked her friends if they knew of anything that could be upsetting her they had no idea, though they agreed that she seemed less than her usual self. I was surprised and rather annoyed that only the science teacher commented on Alice's health when I spoke to the staff at the parents' evening.

During this time the question of Alice moving on to boarding school when she was 16 arose. Beth and Jenny had completed their A levels through the state system at two different schools situated in the city about 15 miles away and, although their sixth-form years had been perfectly satisfactory, I think both the girls would say it was not their favourite spell of education. Alice had always been captivated by the typical 'American chick films' with cheerleaders and glamorous school proms and I had shared with her my very happy memories of moving away to boarding school when I was 16. I was conscious of the fact that Alice was looking at another four years of education without her sisters' company and the nearest bus stop three miles away. It had become apparent as Beth and Jenny progressed through school and as the workload increased that there was less time to see friends after school, particularly when we moved to the farm.

Alice was showing very little enthusiasm for anything at this stage but this idea did seem to catch her imagination.

Ian was curious, too, and so we all went to look at three schools within two hours' drive of home. Alice showed a real interest during the introductory talks and tours of each school but her mood tended to regress once we returned to the privacy of the car. However, one school in particular attracted her, and on that occasion she went home in a good mood and showed more excitement than she had done for a long time.

The next important date in the diary was Beth's twenty-first birthday in February 2001. She decided to have a small dinner party with close friends and godparents to celebrate, and her boyfriend offered to cook for the occasion. It had been six weeks since Beth and Jenny had seen Alice, and I wondered if they would notice a further decline in their sister. They both agreed that she probably was thinner than when they last saw her but the general view was that I was over-worrying and that Alice was just going through a funny phase. I was becoming increasingly frustrated that I couldn't seem to find anyone who could understand what I was concerned about.

It had now been five months since Alice had last had a period, though I wasn't overly concerned because she was comparatively new to a menstrual cycle. However, her weight loss became increasingly obvious, she was drinking copious amounts of water and she continued to be exceptionally quiet. Her behaviour began to concern me: we spent hours in Tesco and she developed a fascination with anything to do with food, such as cooking programmes and recipe books, and took huge pleasure in cooking delicious meals for us, though she declined them herself. We talked a lot and she assured me that everything was fine. However, I was extremely concerned generally and felt that there must be some physical explanation. I suggested that we should go and see the GP. She finally agreed and I was relieved at last to be seeing a professional, who I hoped would find a cause for this worrying situation, and a solution. My fear was that Alice was diabetic, as she had lost weight and was drinking so much – the usual symptoms of diabetes.

The appointment, however, was a disaster. Alice was quiet and unforthcoming, and when asked by the doctor why she was there, she explained that she was worried because she hadn't had a period for five months. I was shocked that without looking at her, he asked if she was pregnant. I explained that Alice was drinking an awful lot of water and I thought she'd lost some weight, and I also described to him the problem we had had with her rigmaroles a few years before. After a urine test, diabetes was ruled out and he suggested that we come back in a couple of months if there was still no sign of a period. However, I was surprised at how he had asked relatively few questions and did not relate well to Alice.

By this time I was becoming increasingly disturbed, frustrated and, quite frankly, irritated. Jenny often came home for weekends to see her boyfriend. She loved cooking and food but Alice always seemed to be hanging around the cooker. If Jenny made a cheese sauce, Alice would be standing there watching with awe as Jenny poured it over a plateful of pasta. Jenny quickly noticed that Alice had not only taken control of her meals but of ours as well and wondered what on earth was going on.

The tension between us all was increasing. Alice was eating completely different meals from the rest of us but her plate was still reasonably full. She vanished into the sitting room and took an age eating her supper, cutting every bit into the tiniest morsels. Ian was becoming more and more angry. If friends came round for supper, Alice would not join in the conversation but lay silently in front of the fire doing her homework, as if waiting for some kind of comment from us all. I found the entire situation acutely embarrassing and I couldn't reconcile everyone's different viewpoints. Nobody else shared the long haul of going up and down the aisles of Tesco looking at different 'Healthy Eating' products, and I didn't want to suggest to Alice that she should do her homework upstairs, out of fear of alienating her further. I shared my doubts with Miranda, my closest friend and Alice's godmother, but she, too, was of the opinion that Alice was simply being a pain and that there was nothing more sinister in it.

The one thing that Ian and I agreed on was that Alice was allowing her social life to lapse. We were surprised on a couple of occasions when Alice phoned us asking to be collected early from parties. She clearly was not embracing the music, drink and boys that her contemporaries were experiencing. She was a forlorn figure in the car park waiting for rescue, with no trace of the fun-loving, quick-witted and confident girl we had seen only a few months before at Ian's party. I was the only person who could see all the familiar aspects of my darling Alice gradually disappearing. It was frustrating that my family, Ian, close friends and, finally, the doctor were largely dismissive of what I felt was a storm brewing. Why Alice was being so difficult I had no idea, but I knew that it wasn't merely an adolescent sulk. Most extraordinarily, at the time, Alice's weight loss seemed almost incidental to all the other characteristics that she was exhibiting.

Shortly before Easter it was obvious to everyone that there was a major problem. Alice was extremely thin. She packed her own lunch for school and was eating smaller portions in the evening. In the mornings she was embarking on a rigorous work-out routine of stomach crunches and press-ups, which she argued was typical of anyone her age who wanted to be fit. I couldn't understand why she went up and down the stairs so often, but she came back with perfectly good excuses for this, too, saying that she needed to collect a book, a pen or a tissue, and so on. She became immersed in her schoolwork and I had a dreadful feeling that her rigmaroles had returned, most noticeably in the form of frantic hand washing. As well as fearing having dirty hands and shoes, she was also anxious about kitchen and bathroom cleaners remaining on her skin. As a result, she washed her hands repeatedly and they were beginning to look sore.

Having had to wear spectacles for a couple of years, Alice had been keen to try contact lenses and she had mastered the art of fitting them very well a few months earlier. However, her contact lenses were now proving to be a problem; each lens was meant to last for a month but they were constantly becoming torn because of the repetitive cleaning with the cleansing solution that Alice felt was necessary to prevent any contamination coming into contact with her eyes.

Finally the penny was beginning to drop, and I phoned the Eating Disorders Association in March. I spoke to a helpful woman there who seemed particularly worried when I mentioned the heavy exercise routine. I remember her saying, 'It does sound like anorexia but I hope it isn't.'

She advised me to take Alice back to the GP and also suggested a couple of books that might be useful: Janet Treasure, *Anorexia Nervosa: A Survival Guide for Families, Friends and Sufferers* and Rachel Bryant-Waugh and Bryan Lask, *Eating Disorders: A Parents' Guide*.

These two books became my bibles for a while and they certainly diagnosed the illness that I had been unable to fathom. They explained the 'anorexic minx' that was controlling Alice's brain and gave me case studies of families going through exactly the same maze. It was extraordinary to discover there in print so many of the abnormalities that I was experiencing reflected by other people, and it represented something of a relief: the withdrawal, the fascination with food in every context except eating it themselves, and the excessive exercise. I read with disbelief the suggested menu plans intended to help the sufferers gain weight, as I knew there was no way in the world that I was going to be able to entice Alice on to the increased-calorie meals suggested. Alice's endless deliberations in Tesco had resulted in an extremely limited diet of tuna fish, pitta bread, baked potatoes, occasionally cottage cheese, and, very rarely, chicken. Milk, cereals, any trace of butter or even fruit had long since been left behind and, although Alice had probably spent in total over an hour looking at different Easter eggs, it was with morbid fascination rather than with any intention of eating one.

About six weeks after the first doctor's appointment we saw a different doctor, who related well to Alice. He was kind, sympathetic and generous with his time. It was the first time anyone had suggested that antidepressants could sometimes be very useful in controlling OCD. But I felt that, at

14, Alice was far too young to be taking such a strong drug and so the antidepressants were not prescribed. The doctor advised me that the eating problems were difficult to tackle and finding the correct plan of action would not be easy, but he offered to see Alice whenever she wanted to talk to him and suggested trying alternative treatments, though Alice had already rejected these. By this time, however, I was frightened and angry with myself for being so stupid as to have let the situation get out of control, but the ball was rolling and I couldn't do a thing to stop it. I spent hours on the phone trying to find someone who could help us, but every time I seemed to hit a brick wall.

A friend gave me a list of counsellors and eventually I found one locally who specialised in OCD and who was prepared to meet and hopefully help Alice with the OCD and her food difficulties. After Alice's first appointment she brought home a diary to record what she was eating each day and I hoped that perhaps I had at last found someone who understood the problems and could resolve them. The counsellor suggested that Alice would feel less inhibited if she met the counsellor on her own, and we booked in for a one-hour weekly session over a period of eight weeks. While I was trying to find professional advice for Alice's condition, the name of a psychiatrist who specialised in adolescent eating disorders kept emerging, either from phone conversations or when looking through lists and directories, but he was affiliated to the local mental health institution and I was still very reluctant to admit that my daughter might have a mental problem.

Finally, Alice's health became too grave to worry about any stigma. I phoned the hospital and asked for an appointment to see the specialist. I was informed that I would have to be referred by my GP and that there was then a six-month waiting list. I was appalled and said that I didn't think I'd have a daughter left to bring in six months' time. I phoned the GP immediately and asked him to write a letter asking for an appointment as quickly as possible. During the ten weeks of waiting for our appointment Alice's health dived. She was frighteningly thin, hardly eating, cold and withdrawn, and she was washing, exercising and working excessively. For me the most agonising part was that Alice would not let me kiss her in case she 'caught' a calorie from me.

I spoke to Alice's counsellor and advised her that I was seeking further professional advice, which I think came as a relief to her; she hadn't realised that once Alice had begun counselling I had not continued taking her to see the GP. I longed for the hospital appointment to arrive because, finally, I felt that we were going to meet someone who could help us.

When I look back on this period of Alice's illness, I often wonder if I could have done things differently and prevented her from sliding so far down the slippery slope. My 'bibles' implied that support was my main role. However, I later read Dee Dawson's book, *Anorexia Nervosa and Bulimia: A Parents' Guide to Recognising Eating Disorders and Taking Control*, which presented a different angle. It suggested that a firm stance was vital. But I had already lost that battle. Quietly and effectively Alice had gained control of her eating habits without too much objection from me. Further reading suggested that non-confrontational parents were more susceptible to having an anorexic child and I certainly fitted into that category. The girls and I had always shared a friendship and mutual respect and I had never had to be the heavy-handed disciplinarian. I didn't believe that getting annoyed with Alice was going to be the answer. Any rows were between Ian and myself concerning our different opinions as to how we should handle Alice. Ian's approach was either to ignore Alice or get cross with her, which I felt only aggravated their already fragile relationship.

In retrospect it is all so painfully obvious that Alice was becoming anorexic, but at the time it was impossible to fit the jigsaw together; there were so many aspects that were unexplainable, but a plausible justification could be found to excuse them all. Although her weight loss was a major part of the equation, her fascination with food had completely thrown me off the scent.

I realise now that I should not have allowed our first visit to the GP to be so unsatisfactory. It had taken considerable persuasion to get Alice there in the first place, and although my fears of diabetes were quickly eliminated I should have pursued an explanation for the symptoms she was manifesting at the time. I will wonder to this day if I made an enormous mistake in not considering the suggestion of anti-depressants to control Alice's OCD and, had they been successful, whether they would have assisted in combating the onslaught of anorexia. Who knows.

I should have made regular appointments with the GP who had sincerely offered his time to Alice. Had he seen Alice every week, he would undoubtedly have soon realised that she needed specialist help. But I had taken the decision that the counsellor was the better qualified to deal with Alice's problems.

By now Alice in Wonderland had disappeared. It is the memory of Alice's eyes that will haunt me for ever: there was absolutely nothing but two dark sockets of misery.

The only familiar part of Alice that still survived was our friendship, but otherwise all her personal characteristics, which had given so much pleasure, had vanished. I had to acquaint myself with this new reflection of Alice in the looking glass.

CHAPTER 2

A Safety Net

On 22 May 2001, one week before Alice's fifteenth birthday, the long-awaited appointment day came for us to meet the specialist. I appreciated later that I was tremendously fortunate that Alice was as eager for the appointment as I was. It was a gruelling afternoon. We were advised that initially Alice would be interviewed by the consultant psychiatrist and a specialist registrar on her own and then I would join her. We were also introduced to a team of experts who, it was explained, would be assessing the interviews through a one-way window.

Alice was ushered into a room and I was asked to remain in the waiting room until I was called. I went outside and smoked a cigarette, absolutely dreading the ordeal that lay ahead and wondering how Alice was coping. The only time I had ever seen a room like that was on television during police interrogation scenes – I had no idea how I was going to cope.

Alice and I met briefly after her interview. She was obviously very upset and we agreed that it was an extremely difficult afternoon. Then it was time for us to make our entry. It was everything I dreaded – and more.

The questions came hard and penetrating, with some of them covering aspects of my life that I had never discussed with Alice and I didn't want her to hear. 'Had your divorce been violent?' came as a thunderbolt. As far as I was aware, Alice had escaped the occasional scene that had erupted during the marital break-up and it was hard admitting that sometimes the odd chair had flown across the kitchen floor. I knew I had to give an honest response to everything that was asked about my relationship with Ian and Beth and Jenny, but I felt totally exposed and inadequate. Within two hours we had packed in our life history and all Alice's problems. It was a traumatic and often unsympathetic afternoon but, nevertheless, I left with the feeling that I could trust these people. We arranged a further meeting in a month's time to review Alice's progress.

After the meeting we met with a dietician who carefully discussed with Alice a suggested new meal plan with increased calorie content. We had arranged a two-week holiday in France before our next appointment, so we were given some guidelines as to what she should eat during that time. It was a small but definite calorie increase and Alice seemed prepared to give it a try.

Before we left for France we received an 'assessment' from the consultant psychiatrist which was also sent to our GP and David. It documented our lives excellently. In two sheets of A4 paper my ideals of bringing up a functioning family were blown to pieces. I was devastated to read in such factual terms this stark analysis of our lives. Although it was accurate, there was absolutely nothing in it to suggest that at any time or any place we had actually been a happy family. No doubt it was a fair reflection of Alice's thoughts at the time but this interpretation made me feel such a failure that my last traces of confidence vanished.

I already knew the holiday in France was going to be a disaster, but I couldn't find a plausible get-out clause. Months before, Ian and I had planned that we would take the car and drive down to our destination. Alice, Jenny and her boyfriend, and Olivia, Luke and his girlfriend would fly out and join us for the first week. The second week was going to be a 'grown-up' week when some close friends would join us. Although we had confirmation of Alice's illness, my and Ian's family were insistent that Alice's problems should not be allowed to spoil our plans. The professionals had not suggested that Alice was too unwell to travel, so I was left with no excuse other than to continue the holiday as scheduled.

The view among family and friends was that we should have a break and that it might do everyone the world of good. I thought I would scream if anyone repeated that phrase one more time. I knew I would be there to protect Alice for the first week but the second week was going to be disastrous. My friend Miranda and Beth both very innocently offered to fill the gap: Miranda was happy to have Alice stay for four nights and Beth offered to come home for the last weekend to look after her. I warned them both that it would be a difficult task and left them with a long list of instructions and ingredients, which I hoped that Alice would follow.

Alice had a terrible battle during her week's holiday. She was freezing cold in the South of France and spent what little time was left after arguments wrapped up in towels after demented lengths in the pool. Every mealtime was a row, and we were not managing the new meal plan that the dietician had set. Jenny was livid, Luke and his girlfriend completely uninterested. Olivia spent a lot of the time on her mobile phone to her new boyfriend and Ian looked forward to the second week of adult company. Alice 'celebrated' her fifteenth birthday at a restaurant with the arrival of a sparkler-lit birthday cake. Cutting the cake was easy; cutting the atmosphere was impossible. Most of all I dreaded the day when Alice was due to leave – how was she possibly going to manage the week ahead with Miranda and Beth? I wept when she left. Although Ian was sympathetic, he never suggested that I get on a plane and go home. My anguish was tremendous and I dreaded the prospect of attempting another week's holiday.

During that second week Beth and Miranda came to understand just how ill Alice was and they finally appreciated that I had not been dealing with rational behaviour. Miranda's husband Roger had spent four days eating more than he had ever eaten in his life in an attempt to encourage Alice to eat something, and when they saw Alice in her pyjamas Miranda phoned me to say that she thought Alice was going to die if I didn't get a grip on the situation very soon. Beth phoned in tears because she was completely unable to follow the meal plan or control Alice's exercise. Eventually Ian and I drove home; we'd had a break but it hadn't done us any good. It was an agonising way to gain appreciation of the severity of our problems.

Before our holiday in France I informed Alice's school that she was suffering from anorexia and was unwell. However, since her work had continued to be of a high standard the staff did not show much concern. Shortly after the holiday Alice was due to begin two weeks' work experience assisting teaching staff during lessons in her old primary school. I tried to dissuade her from attempting this, but no to avail, and eventually I contacted a member of staff at the school, whom I knew, to explain about Alice's illness and ask her to check that Alice ate a cereal bar at breaktime. Alice was adamant that she would be able to cope and so I agreed on the condition that I would meet her every lunchtime so that I could be with her while she ate her lunch in the car.

It was the most surreal time. Each day I dropped off a child whose appearance was appalling; each night she came home exhausted, but she had completed the work experience. However, it was obvious that she was too unwell to return to school and, much to her anger, I informed her tutor that Alice would not be returning that term. Life at home was utterly bizarre when we were at home together. Mealtimes were a nightmare, and Alice became increasingly argumentative over every ingredient and quantity of food she had agreed to eat. The suggested menu was:

1 glass of water before breakfast
Breakfast
60g cereal
150ml semi-skimmed milk
200ml orange juice plus 100ml water
1 packet raisins mixed with the cereal
strawberries on top of the cereal
1 glass of water after breakfast

Lunch
½ pitta bread
1 teaspoon tuna

1 small apple
1 glass of water

Snack
1 low-fat yogurt or ¾ Nutrigrain bar
200ml orange juice plus 100ml water
1 glass of water

1 glass of water before supper

Supper
small main course
200ml fruit juice plus 100ml water

However, it was impossible for her to eat even this small menu. She drank the water, but otherwise it was a lost cause. One teaspoon of tuna fish was far too variable: which teaspoon was I using to measure the tuna? Strawberries on top of the cereal – not really; maybe one, but the scales were weighing the cereal incorrectly, and certainly the idea of even touching a milk bottle was repellent, let alone the suggestion of actually pouring some into a bowl. The deliberations over the varying yogurts available at Tesco were endless; the store was completely unreasonable in offering only 9,648 types of yogurt and not the 9,649th that would have been suitable. And as for a small main course, forget it, a small main course was invisible according to Alice – and so it went on and on.

Her rigmaroles were becoming more and more apparent. Her hands were red-raw from repeated washing and it was taking her longer and longer to manage her contact lenses. An odd new feature also began to make an appearance before she could even begin to sit down and attempt to eat a meal: she had to complete a small series of jumps on the spot. Usually she was spared the anxiety of anyone seeing this, but there was no stopping her even if a friend or her sisters were watching with disbelief. Miranda witnessed it one evening and decided to mimic Alice and her jumps. It was awful at the time, but almost in embarrassed relief the three of us laughed as Miranda bounced around the place.

By now I felt completely numb. My brain simply could not come to terms with the horrendous decline that it was being asked to decipher. Just nine months before, Alice had been a healthy, normal girl. Now she had lost almost 30 per cent of her body weight and was unrecognisable, not only in appearance but in her personality, too. By the time our family and friends realised that the storm I had warned was brewing had finally broken, I had built a kind of protective barrier around Alice and we were isolated in the tormented world that I had allowed her to create. Although I knew Alice was dictating all our lives, it never crossed my mind to change my engulfing allegiance to her.

We had been having two-weekly appointments with the specialist team for two months since our return from France, and Alice also met Sarah, a charge nurse at the unit, to begin motivational enhancement therapy where the dangers of the illness were explained and Alice could talk about her feelings and perceptions. It was during these sessions with Sarah that Alice could express the concerns she had about her body image, though I do not know exactly what they discussed. However, by mid-June the question of admitting Alice to the unit had arisen. She was, unsurprisingly, strongly against the idea. We also met the family therapist, and Ian joined me for a further appointment with him. It was a stressful meeting with some difficult questions, and Ian was heated in his answers. He had borne the brunt of my outbursts at home; although he had done what he could to help, I had increasingly withdrawn from his company and he was angry about the lack of involvement from Alice's father. He was not prepared to participate in any further meetings because he disliked the sessions and the therapist. My thoughts sunk still further.

Alice was given a far more rigid meal plan, and every item on her plate or in a glass needed to be weighed or measured. The consultant suggested that she should do nothing more strenuous than a short stroll. Behind the instructions I remember him quietly offering the facility of a 'safety net' should we not succeed at home, but I think my brain had almost blanked out at this point.

I had no success with this new meal plan. Even though I had stopped work, it was impossible to keep an eye on Alice for every minute of every day, so limiting her exercise was impossible. I slowly realised that even her voice had vanished as she disappeared yet again up and down the stairs. But she was always there to do the hay and the watering, skipping and jumping over the paddocks and gates, an image that should reflect the antics of an exuberant child rather than the agonised soul that Alice had become. Even if I believed that I had curtailed her exercise regime in the morning, no doubt her alarm clock had been set earlier.

Three events have stayed with me. Jenny was home for the summer. She had completed her first year at university and she decided to confront Alice with the symptoms of anorexia nervosa after another fraught episode by the cooker. The list was endless: preoccupation with food, spending long periods of time reading cookery books, very restricted eating, preference for eating alone, cooking meals for the family, choosing low-calorie foods to the exclusion of anything else, irritability, distress and arguing, strange behaviour around food such as cutting it into small pieces, excessive exercising, wearing baggy clothes, increased activities unrelated to food such as homework, social withdrawal, loss of periods, dizziness, marked tendency to feel the cold, development of fine downy hair. Jenny proved her point, and Alice left the room. I knew that Jenny adored her sister but was finding Alice's behaviour increasingly intolerable. She had a physically demanding summer ahead, working for long hours on the farm cutting celery to finance her through another year at university. I dreaded the prospect of an antagonistic summer between the two sisters. So, to avoid further disruption, I suggested that Jenny stay with her boyfriend for the rest of the summer.

The second event was on my birthday, 19 June 2001. Miranda phoned while she was on holiday to see how we were getting on. 'Not well' was the reply. When she asked how Alice was I simply broke down in tears, and I explained that it was looking increasingly likely that Alice would be admitted to the unit. Miranda was as dumbfounded as I had first been when told that the average period of admission was four months.

My last memory of Alice before her admission is of a Saturday afternoon when Olivia and her boyfriend phoned to see if they could take her punting. It was a kind thought; they knew Alice was meant to have as little exercise as possible but they had hoped that it would at least provide a change of scene for her. They returned about three hours later. Alice was exhausted, cold, dizzy and frightened, I think, by her own frailty. She fell asleep in my arms. I was terrified. I thought she was going to die, and phoned up the hospital asking for the 'safety net' as soon as possible.

On 5 July 2001 Alice was admitted to hospital, though not as an inpatient as I had believed would be the case. The consultant explained that it would be a mistake to move her straight to inpatient treatment. He felt that if she were admitted as an inpatient she might find it particularly difficult to return home again, because of its association with her fears and rigmaroles. In any case, they did not have a bed available at that time. And so Alice attended the unit seven days a week, from 7.30 a.m. until 7.30 p.m. including all meals; it was fortuitous that we lived within 20 miles of a specialist adolescent eating disorders unit.

Ian drove us to the hospital that first morning. I deeply hoped that there was still enough of the old Alice to see her through the next difficult period of her life. I advised her to try to find the more 'positive' patients and to give it her best – and with a huge hug I left her. I was extremely upset but relieved that I had passed over the responsibility of Alice's care to the professionals.

CHAPTER 3

Jumping into Oblivion

Welcome to Planet Anorexia. The next few months were going to see Alice on a one-way ticket to hell, with her family in a totally alien environment that was incomprehensible, destructive and exhausting. My solace was that I was going to meet other families who were experiencing the same trip.

The eating disorders unit was unlike any hospital I had ever seen. It was difficult to distinguish between the staff and family, but not the 'patients'. The atmosphere was extraordinary: it seemed ghostly quiet except for the continual background noise of the television. After a couple of weeks I had become accustomed to the structure and routines of the unit and appreciated how fortunate Alice was to be in the hands of such exceptional care.

The first extraordinary part of the journey for me was phoning Alice in the early afternoon of her first day in the unit. Her familiar quiet voice answered the phone. I asked her how she was doing, and after a little while she whispered that she had eaten a sandwich and yogurt for lunch. I asked her how she had managed this and she simply replied, 'I had to.' I couldn't believe it; I had spent the past month coercing

Alice to eat a quarter of a piece of bread with a teaspoon of tuna fish with no success.

My job was to collect Alice every evening at about 7.45 p.m., put her to bed, wake her in the morning and get her back to the unit before breakfast at 8.00 a.m. It sounded so simple; if meals were taken out of the equation, surely I could manage this much of her life.

Alice came home the first night and seemed to accept the new regime surprisingly well. She was the only outpatient out of the group of ten children and was relieved to be coming home for the night. She had eaten her three meals but was extremely agitated that she was not allowed to go on the twice-daily 20-minute walk with fellow patients. She described her day, which included three meals, one-hour quiet time after she completed each meal, a morning and evening meeting to discuss issues arising during the day, and school from 10.00 a.m. until 4.00 p.m. We actually had the bulk of the conversation while we went for a walk after she got home. She ran up and down the stairs quite a few times and skipped along the corridor, but when I tucked her into bed I was optimistic that she would follow the programme.

Beth's graduation was scheduled during Alice's first week. It was a 400-mile round trip to the university in Liverpool. I was so absorbed with Alice that I didn't think I could really fit this into an already tight schedule. Ian quietly pointed out that this was a big day for Beth and that we should be there. It was a happy day and I will always be grateful that Ian insisted that we went. However, Alice was angry that we were an hour late collecting her and did not ask anything about our day.

The first weekend at the unit was difficult. Some of the children who were making progress were allowed home with their families. Alice and the newer arrivals remained there, but their families were allowed to visit. I had not been involved with any of Alice's meals at this stage and it seemed easiest if I came to see her after lunch. I understood that Alice was meant to be sitting down as much as possible and I tried to think of an activity that she might enjoy, so I dug out some old photographs and hoped that together we could put them in an album. She couldn't have been less interested and was extremely restless. I noticed that some of the other children were sitting quietly reading or doing cross-stitch, and wondered how on earth Alice was going to adapt. She had never been a child who had enjoyed puzzles or games, though she had certainly watched some television in her time.

I left Alice while she had her supper and went to have a cup of coffee in Tesco until it was time to collect her. I felt extraordinarily lonely and hoped that she would be in a reasonable mood when I collected her. She was extremely relieved to leave the unit. On her return home we walked and talked and she skipped and jumped her way to bed.

I planned to do a repeat of Saturday's visit on Sunday – arriving after lunch again – but this time I substituted painting for the photos. Again it was a failure and Alice was becoming increasingly unhappy. Tears began to flow, and she whispered that she was simply not going to be able to cope with the new restrictions put upon her.

The family therapist arranged weekly appointments, and Beth and Jenny offered to attend whenever they could. Alice's initial contribution to the meetings was minimal. She sat hunched on a chair, head down and arms crossed, while Jenny, Beth and I tried to make some kind of a conversation with the therapist. It became apparent quite quickly that the two sisters were going to have different approaches to Alice's illness. Jenny was the strongest and most willing to confront Alice on her behaviour whereas Beth and I took a gentler attitude. It was going to prove a useful combination. The family therapist was sympathetic towards Alice and I remember him emphasising how tired Alice must be. Although I was prepared to participate in the meetings, deep down I was finding it difficult to accept that I now needed the help of a therapist to manage my family. It took quite a few appointments before I realised that the therapist was providing invaluable assistance towards helping us to learn how to manage Alice's illness.

I approached the second week apprehensively. Although Alice did not put up much protest at the prospect of another week, she was reluctant to go. She was particularly fearful about having to be weighed on the Tuesday. The week did not go well; Alice did not put on the required amount of weight and was furious that her meal plan (in other words, calories) was increased. She couldn't leave the unit quickly enough in the evenings and this was no doubt because I could not maintain the same activity restrictions at home. Alice's skipping was beginning to be replaced by jumping. This was the beginning of the nightmare I could never have dreamed of, and which would continue to frighten me even more than the starvation.

Within a very short period of Alice's admission I had evacuated our home. Alice's calories had increased each week but her weight had not. I told Ian that I would be unable to cook our supper each evening and asked him to stay away. I didn't want anyone to see what Alice and I were experiencing. Her jumping had escalated to such extremes that it is nearly impossible to describe. Initially I thought it was random behaviour, but as time went on I came to realise that it was completely ritualised and Alice would not allow anything to interfere or interrupt it. Everything from putting on a sock to stepping out of the door required its own peculiar series of jumps.

Our mornings began at 5.45 a.m. I needed to be on the road by 7.15 to get Alice to the unit by eight o'clock. On waking she immediately embarked on a strenuous work-out. As each separate item of clothing went on, another series of jumps was completed. Every action — brushing teeth, brushing hair, moving from one room to another — demanded another set of jumps. It was taking her about five minutes to fit her contact lenses because there were so many different jumps and different hand-washing rituals that had to be completed between each lens. Downstairs each kitchen drawer had to be kicked six times. Before I could coax Alice into the car we had to go on a ten-minute walk. On our arrival at the hospital she vanished to the loo and completed another exhaustive work-out. I can remember so clearly standing outside the loo door and begging her to come out. I never saw any staff during these episodes but I knew the receptionist must be hearing what was going on and, once again, I felt so ridiculously useless that I was unable to control Alice. I eventually managed to deliver her to the care of the staff at the unit.

As soon as I collected Alice from the unit at 7.45 p.m. the routines would begin again. Once in the car she immediately began leg exercises, and, although she was strapped in the car, she continually tried to lift herself out of the seat. When we arrived home at about 8.30 she jumped in and out of the door six times, kicked all the kitchen drawers, ran up the stairs, skipped and touched the ceiling and jumped before she went to the bathroom, where she washed her hands again and again. After that she ran out into the garden, and jumped over the gates and fences to see the horses.

After about the first two weeks at the unit Alice had been allowed to participate in some exercise. It was strictly regulated to two 20-minute walks a day with a member of staff, but when she was at home she begged me to take her for a short walk. I knew it was in complete contradiction of the rules set by the unit, but I hoped that in some way it would relieve some of the tension. It was the only part of the day I had with Alice when she was in some kind of control and we could make an attempt at a conversation. I suggested that she help me water the garden, because I thought it would kill some time and it would not allow her the opportunity to jump, but whenever my back was turned she was hiding round the corner jumping with the hosepipe in her hand, watering the road.

The next prolonged stage was getting Alice to bed. Each discarded article of clothing required its own jumping or hand-washing ritual. She jumped while she brushed her teeth, and removing her contact lenses in the evening was as difficult as it had been in the morning. The jumps continued while she got into the bath and while she was bathing, and then she went into an astonishing work-out to mark getting out of the bath. Every possible variation of jump was demonstrated. With a spectacular grand finale, she allowed herself to jump exhausted into bed. The process of Alice getting to bed was taking over two and a half hours.

The staff at the unit, too, were aware that Alice was experiencing difficulties in controlling her rituals, as they had seen her jumping throughout the day.

Most evenings I came downstairs and had a glass or two of wine, listened to some music and cried. I was completely bewildered and was forced to come to terms with the fact that Alice had, for the time being, lost the plot. She was not functioning 'normally' in any respect.

I suppose Ian was the only person who had an inkling of what was going on, because on some mornings he took us to the hospital and on others he drove us home. He asked her to try to sit quietly in the car because it was unsafe to drive with so much movement in the back. He also witnessed Alice kicking the kitchen drawers and jumping before she put her shoes on, and jumping again before she could step out of the back door.

I frequently spoke to my mother on the phone but really it was impossible for anyone else to begin to understand the full horror of the situation. My feeling of isolation by now was enormous and I could not begin to explain to family and friends just how out of control Alice and I were.

In retrospect I realise that it was extraordinary that I didn't disclose the enormity of the problems I was experiencing to the professionals. Perhaps it was a combination of factors that prevented this. Since my divorce I had become very protective and defensive of the children. I was unable to admit that I was not managing the simple requirements the unit had set and also I knew from her incidents at home that Alice would condemn me if I were to critise her behaviour in any way.

At the same time Alice provided me with a keyhole. She said in passing that she would love to receive post in the mornings as some of the inpatients did. I popped a card in the letterbox and, by hand, I received from Alice a letter expressing more than she had disclosed for a long time. It was the first of many desperate letters I was to receive, and it was the beginning of a vital point of contact. During the next couple of months our letters became our lifeline. We could both express on paper things that we avoided in direct conversation. We congratulated each other on our successes, and apologised for our mistakes. Alice wrote frankly, doubting her sanity. It was an extraordinary contradiction, because her letters were so completely sane. On 25 July 2001 she wrote:

> *I'm not convinced I'm really getting anywhere. I just want to be the way I used to be, what happened to me – what did I do to deserve this . . . do you think my brain will ever work normally again? I miss thinking normally – isn't that a bizarre thing to say! If anyone were to read our letters they would instantly realise how crazy I was and run as far as they possibly could! (Not that I'd blame them – I seem to put such a strain on people's lives at the moment) . . .*

I chose to ignore the 'green mush' (as we used to describe the anorexic part of Alice's brain), and wrote to 'Pinky' (the nickname we gave to the part of Alice's brain that I knew and loved and that Alice was trying to find again). In time Alice extended this form of communication to friends and family. She also had her 'black book'; I dreaded the times when she insisted that she be left alone to write down her thoughts, and it is still an immensely private book.

By now Alice was receiving cognitive therapy, which is a form of psychotherapy that treats emotional disorders by changing negative patterns of thought. She didn't tell me a great deal about these sessions but I knew that these were the only appointments that Alice looked forward to. She told me that they were humorous and it was obviously a relief for her to meet someone who understood her rigmaroles.

Twelve days after Alice's admission Alice, Beth and I met the team for a 'review meeting'. Everyone immediately connected with Alice's treatment and care was present: the consultant psychiatrist, family therapist, cognitive therapist, staff nurse and teacher from the unit. Alice was quiet but expressed the opinion that she was making progress. As described by the consultant, 'Alice's general demeanour is very pleasant. She is eager to please and polite and friendly. However, it is apparent that there is another side to Alice, which is more angry, determined and resentful. Mrs Kingsley and Beth have both commented how difficult it is to manage with Alice in the period after she returns home at night. It is as though Alice has bottled up all the behaviours during the day and then the cork comes out at night. It is obviously difficult for Alice and her family that she is a day patient. We have therefore discussed the possibility of her being an inpatient. I repeat that although this would provide some short-term relief, I think it very likely that Alice would find it increasingly difficult to return home the longer she stayed here. We agreed that so long as it is bearable, it is better to continue with the current plan of Alice spending days at the unit and returning home at night. We will, of course, need to keep this under review and being an inpatient does remain a possibility.'

From the first day of Alice's admission I decided that my role was to be positive and supportive to her in every way. I tried to walk into the unit with a smile, which probably disguised the agonising start to our mornings and my fearful anticipation of what lay ahead in the evenings. Before any meetings with either the consultant or the family therapist, Alice begged me not to say anything that would in any way contradict her opinion of how she was doing: 'You promise you'll stick up for me Mum, won't you.' Her letters reiterated everything she said:

> . . . never question whether or not you are helping me – every day you keep me going and I hope that you're able not to give up on me. I need you so much, I need you to stick up for me, you're my bestest friend in the entire world, I love you more and more each day and I am so proud you are on my team. Please be on my team tomorrow . . . please don't join the fight against Alice. I know you're not. But I think we both have seen that it works better when we're together and if we are both listening and compromising with one another . . . I'm trying to apply myself more wholeheartedly and I really need your help.

My overwhelming fear was that if I disclosed everything that was happening at home I would alienate Alice. I felt that Alice was testing me in some way and I was not going to fail that test. I knew that some anorexic children could completely shun their parents, and I felt that at least this was one devastation I had managed to avoid.

Alice was sharing some of her innermost thoughts in her letters, and I hoped that we were building a new kind of trust. But I know now that behind my actions to support her was the most natural emotion: my maternal instinct to love and protect my child. This powerful emotion obliterated any idea in my mind that perhaps Alice was manipulating me so that she could continue with her obsessive behaviour.

The combination of these factors no doubt inhibited me from giving a fair reflection of our experiences at home to the team during our appointments. Both Beth and Jenny had noticed this and found my approach exasperating. Although they continued to offer their time and contribute where they could, Beth was the least accessible because she had begun her new career in marketing, 200 miles away. Jenny, however, was the most available while she spent her summer working in the celery fields. Ian, more than either of the girls, knew what was happening at home but as he did not want to be involved with the meetings at the hospital he did not know how I avoided being honest about how bad it was at home.

And so began another of the problems I was going to have to consider: divided loyalties. We all shared the same goal but we were in different camps.

The unit offered me the opportunity to meet up with other parents of anorexic patients on a fortnightly basis during meetings that were arranged to help parents understand the illness. I was initially reluctant to attend these meetings, as I was fearful that I was going to meet the reason for Alice's anorexia: parents. And I did meet parents, parents just like me who loved their children, who had the same stories, same bewilderment and embarrassed relief that finally their daughter or son was in hospital care. Finally I had found an environment where I met kindred spirits and we could share our experiences of Planet Anorexia.

Another concept that sent my brain into panic mode was the 'family meals' offered by the unit. I initially thought I would be asked to join Alice and her fellow inpatients around a table for lunch or supper, but, in fact, the reality turned out to be more frightening. Alice and I were expected to eat our meal in a private room, and I was given the task of measuring Alice's meal as I had attempted to do before her admission. My hands shook as I spread some Flora on her sandwich – a supportive nurse monitored my progress all the time. I fumbled my way through weighing the food, which had seen so many arguments before Alice's admission. I was petrified and felt so stupid; how could I possibly have lost so much confidence that I was frozen while preparing a simple meal for my child? We were offered every possible support during the meal, and it was agreed that a nurse would look in every ten minutes to check that all was well. As Alice asked that we never spoke about food during the meal, we took in the radio to fill in any silences. We got through the meal, though Alice was able to convince me that I could break one or two rules set by the unit such as finding a small spoon for her cereal and pouring her an extra glass of water. Nonetheless, she ate her food and I was euphoric.

After Alice had remained in the unit seven days a week for a month I was allowed to take her out for a day, including a meal. It was a welcome relief for Alice. Her days at the unit seemed to last even longer than before since the schoolwork in the hospital had finished for the summer holiday. She was so excited and I was so nervous. We agreed that I would make a cottage cheese sandwich. Alice assured me that a ' "Healthy Eating" cottage cheese would be fine – nobody's parents make a sandwich with ordinary cottage cheese.' I complied. I prayed that Saturday, 'Please God, let Alice eat her sandwich,' which is not my usual approach. I played my Tina Turner CD while I prepared the picnic – she has always given me a boost. I tried to make everything look pretty and packed our lunch in a big basket. I planned to take Alice to the races, as she couldn't walk too far and I hoped that she would enjoy seeing the people and horses.

Alice was thrilled at the prospect of a day out of the unit. I was apprehensive but shared her excitement at a glimpse of normality. My first mistake was the big picnic basket. Alice was appalled at the size of it. How much food was I expecting her to eat? First lesson learnt: pack everything into as tiny a package as possible. Alice found it difficult to eat her picnic in the car park – she had to go through her routine of jumps before and during her meal – but she ate it all, and when I returned her to the unit for supper that night I thought we'd had a successful day. She had enjoyed and appreciated it all. God had answered my prayers: Alice had eaten her lunch, and she had mostly managed to control her jumping in a public environment. We had probably walked too far but we had managed a day having fun.

During this period Alice disclosed very little about the thoughts she shared with either Sarah during motivational therapy or during cognitive therapy. The only feedback I had was from her letters, which did not relate directly to either of them. It was a defining moment when Alice showed me a letter that she had written, as part of her motivational therapy, to her *enemy* the anorexic minx, and a second to her *friend*, the anorexic minx. Alice wrote the first letter quite easily, but it was more arduous for her to write the second. She showed me her first letter as soon as she had written it – here was Pinky again. The second letter didn't come to light until months later.

28th July

Dear Anorexia, my enemy,

The deepest, darkest hole I've ever fallen down. Today should be the first day of my summer holidays. Hooray, long sleep in, morning TV, going out with my friends, going out, having a break. About 6 months ago I was so excited – I had so many plans and my God, I was 'having fun'.

But now I've got a very different view of summer holidays. Because of you I'm stuck in hospital, where I'm constantly told to sit down and where I'm always watched because you took away my own sense of control.

I want you out of my life forever and I never, ever want you to torture my brain again. You've taken everything away from me. What did I do which made me need to be punished so cruelly?

I miss my friends so much. I haven't seen them for over 5 weeks. I hate the way you make Mum look so exhausted and so her life revolves around you, why are you so selfish, not only are you breaking me but everyone around me as well – please leave them alone.

I don't understand when you grew so big and your ugly sharp hands took grasp of my entire life – when will you ever let go TOTALLY? For so long I'd be moving along fine, but slowly you restricted my diet and eventually left me starving (apparently to death).

Now I can't eat what I want to eat, I can't eat how much I want to eat and you've made it so hard just simply to eat. And why make me exercise so obsessively, why make me feel so guilty? Why can't I just go to the loo, or get into bed without jumping.

I HATE YOU.

I want my eyes back, my old eyes which were happy in

my body, which didn't analyse every other girl and use them as a comparison to me. I want to look at something and think . . . aawww that looks good, why don't you have some.

But, oh I forgot, you've taken them as well. I'm so sick of being in this room, I'm so sick of this routine. Do you know that in the morning I'm no longer excited about my day? I dread it and it never ends.

By the way, I've been elected sports captain at school – what I've dreamt of since Year 7. I couldn't play netball tomorrow and not just because I wouldn't be allowed to but because even though it's impossible for me to admit I couldn't physically do it.

I've got so many plans for my future, short and long term and I'm going to do every single one. 'Revenge is so sweet.' My revenge to you taking so much of my time is that I will succeed in all my dreams.

I know when you let go, you'll go to hell. But you've broken so many wings. Now we're going to fly again and every day we get a step closer.

Goodbye, forever.

Alice.

And here is the second letter:

Dear Anorexia my Friend,

It has taken me so long to start this letter to you and I don't know whether it's because I don't want to admit that you could be a friend or something I need because I can't understand how you could take so much from me yet still be a friend.

What do you give me?

You give me the power to keep myself thin. I like being thin and I hate the fact that I can't be both better and look the way I do. (Although at times I think I don't like the way I look but yet I'm worried that if I do put on weight issues will always play on my mind.) Being thin means in a way being vulnerable. I don't want to be completely independent and you give me a reason to make sure that others won't just leave me and expect me to survive on my own. But again I don't understand why it is I think people will leave me on my own. I trust Mum and all my family and that they love me for what I am and not just because I have this which makes me fragile.

Reading what I wrote about looking the way I look now seems to unconsciously alarm me – I don't know how I want to look and although I don't feel able to put how I feel into one sentence, I mean, I feel as though you stop me growing up too fast and I don't know how to say it, all my feelings seem to argue against each other. One side fights so hard for you and the other fights for me.

I wonder what new solutions I would have to make if I lost you immediately. I can't see any – without you I'm free to make a decision according to how I feel but with you my day follows a structure. I wonder whether this structure stops me from thinking about things which frighten me – what those things are is a mystery to me.

I like to know people are looking out for me, being the 'baby' of the family.

I seem to enjoy when our friends ask how I'm doing and at times I like hearing when they say I look very thin and they're worried about me. But this isn't the Alice I remember, trying to always show everyone I'm fine and trying my hardest never to stick out or be different.

Being different isn't what you give me; you give me being special. I don't want to be forgotten and I don't want to have lived my life never making an effect upon anyone or never leaving footprints anywhere.

But yet I want to be remembered with a smile upon my face, not tears on my cheeks. I need to decide which I want more – you and your thinness or life and its decisions.

Although no-one believes me, I choose life. Please don't feel betrayed and stay with me as a punishment and please don't swarm someone else's thought.

I think you need to be at peace with yourself too. Good Luck.

Alice

We continued with Alice attending the unit as a day patient for approximately two months. Although her calories were increased each week, she did not gain anything even close to the desired target weight of 1.5kg a week. In fact her weight had increased by only 1.1kg during the whole period, and it was becoming apparent to everyone involved that Alice, rather than making progress, had in many respects deteriorated.

Although Ian continued to reject the counselling services provided by the unit, he tried to help where he could with driving us to the unit and being flexible about my working hours at the farm. Indeed, he recognised much of the anguish that Alice was suffering from the memories of his own nervous breakdown. However, he was becoming increasingly frustrated with my way of tackling Alice's problems, and felt that I should discipline her more. He suggested that I should not allow her to go upstairs until it was time for bed, for example, but although it was a fair suggestion I dismissed it out of hand because I knew I would never be able to implement it.

Jenny was finding the summer difficult, too. Sometimes she would have loved to come home after a long day's work, have a chat and some supper, but instead we met only when we were driving to and from the hospital for another appointment. Unfortunately, I have an awful feeling that in those car rides our conversations revolved around Alice rather than how Jenny's summer was going.

By this time the word had travelled through the grapevine that our home was in turmoil, and so the phone rarely rang. I was relieved – it was so much easier not having to explain.

CHAPTER 4
Out of Our Depth

Over the next four weeks Alice became increasingly abusive, devious and manipulative. We were both exhausted and frightened, and we both dreaded the jumping and washing routines that she had to complete each night and morning. As well as the jumping routines, Alice had taken to vomiting. She told the consultant that it happened spontaneously and was not under her control, though she sometimes swallowed it and sometimes spat it out. She was sick before she got into the car, as soon as she got out of the car, in the garden, in the kitchen and in the bathroom. She made no secret of it. Even at the unit Alice would spontaneously vomit in the wastepaper basket or flowerpot without a second thought. Her pockets were filled with tissues containing assorted fragments of food, which she had managed to remove from her meals without anyone noticing. Undoubtedly this, too, contributed to her failure to gain weight. The unit continued to watch her carefully and supervise her visits to the loo.

The consultant suggested that we should set a timetable for the evenings with the hope of controlling the jumping: sitting and watching television for an hour when we got home, five minutes getting ready for a bath, 20 minutes in the bath, and so on, until bed. But just as with the increased meal plans that Alice had agreed to before her admission, once in the privacy of our home Alice totally refused to cooperate. There was absolutely no chance that I would be able to persuade her to sit down for an hour watching television and I completely failed to implement even one aspect of the timetable.

Beth offered to come home for a weekend to give me a break. She was appalled at Alice's deterioration since the last time she had been home, and watched and heard with horror Alice refuting every attempt I made to stop her jumping and stick to the new regime. However, she was confident that she could cope with Alice for one evening and suggested that Ian and I should go out for supper with friends. It was a wonderful gesture, but halfway through the evening I received a phone call from her beseeching us to come home. When I arrived home Beth and Alice were hysterical from their arguments and the house was upside down. Although the weekend was a disaster for Beth, for me it was such a relief to have her there and sharing Alice's and my anguish. Beth had no suggestions and no criticisms, but she quietly took the nightmare on board.

One weekend the unit allowed Alice and me to have breakfast at home, but I had tremendous apprehension about preparing the meal, knowing that we would not have the support of the unit. By this time my kitchen cupboard contained assorted scales, all of which, for one reason or another, Alice had found fault with. So I made another purchase, the exact replica of the scales at the unit. I prepared everything the night before. It took a long time: the weighing of food, measuring of drinks, level teaspoon of

Flora and level teaspoon of marmalade, the clingfilm, the agreed bowls, plates and glasses. The unit had removed raisins from Alice's meal plan, substituting two apples, because she was so adept at hiding them; I agreed that as a treat she could have raisins at home. It took her a long time to eat her breakfast and it irritated her that she had a far bigger breakfast than me. I found the raisins later.

After about six weeks I could join Alice on her walks without a member of staff accompanying us if I was there at the correct time. We walked vast distances at an incredible pace with Alice criss-crossing the road and jumping on and off the curb throughout, but she always assured me that this was a typical outing. I knew I was being taken advantage of, but I was terrified that if I tackled her too firmly on the subject she would run off and I would lose sight of her altogether.

I followed Alice for every minute that she was 'in my care', and tried to encourage and control her. Although the books I had been reading implied that making the child feel guilty was counter-productive, sometimes frustration got the better of me and I lost my temper. One evening Alice attacked me for never eating any supper and I attacked her in return, asking how there could possibly be any time for supper when she was incapable of getting herself into the bath and to bed. I slammed the bathroom door and left her to her own devices. I listened for more than an hour while she jumped and struggled to get herself to bed. For the first time ever we didn't make friends that night. It was becoming increasingly difficult to say the right thing: if I praised Alice for a tiny victory she would retort 'Don't say well done!' and then 20 minutes later I would be reprimanded for not congratulating her on a different achievement.

One morning we were late leaving for the unit. Alice had taken longer than ever to get ready and there was no time for her customary ten-minute walk. I insisted that she get in the car. I thought I'd won a battle until we arrived at the hospital grounds. Alice opened the car door while I was still driving and jumped out. She vanished and I met her 20 minutes later. I remember meeting her at the unit and saying, 'If you ever do that again, I will wring your scraggy little neck.' A staff nurse came out of the loo just in time to hear my speech. I was so ashamed.

During this time the amount of punishment Alice's tiny body could absorb was unbelievable: her hands were red-raw from the endless washing and her ankles and feet were becoming increasingly swollen. I asked her to show them to the doctor and received a letter from Alice explaining that the doctor thought the problem was 'because my bones stick out so much and that my skin is very fragile'. How stupid of me not to speak to the doctor myself; I doubt that Alice ever showed her ankles to anyone. She also had a suspiciously large sore towards the base of her spine, which looked rather like a bedsore. Although she assured me that once she was in bed she fell asleep, I am sure that during the night she embarked on another work-out, which would have explained the bruising. As she continued her frenzied routines I wondered just how much pain she was enduring. At the time she totally dismissed it, but much later she admitted that it had been agonising for her.

Alice and I had continued going out on Saturdays for picnics, but I was finding them increasingly difficult. I knew how to prepare the food but was losing the exercise battle. We always walked for miles, though at least Alice mostly managed to control her jumping when in public. The family therapist wanted us to make a strategy on our days out to retrieve some kind of order, and Alice reluctantly agreed that I would return her to the unit at four o'clock rather than six o'clock. The first Saturday I implemented this new regime was a nightmare. Alice was disgusting all day and spoke some of the cruellest words she could muster, but because I knew a schedule had been set I was not going to allow her to break it. We returned to the unit at four o'clock in tears and not speaking to each other. It was the first time I found myself weeping at the unit. I left Alice to have her supper and had another spell in Tesco dreading our trip home. Amazingly, when I collected her, Alice's mood had passed – we had managed to control a situation and, perhaps, new parameters were set.

The unit suggested that we should attempt to lead as normal a life as possible, and when Alice was at home I decided to ask Miranda and Roger over for supper. They knew we were experiencing tremendous problems and understood it might not be an easy evening. I didn't tell Alice until we were driving home, and her behaviour confirmed my worst nightmares. She refused to go into the house – how could she do her usual routine with people watching her? Our friends sat patiently in the sitting room while Alice and I went out for a walk, but on our return they heard Alice angrily shouting abuse at me, slamming doors and tearfully refusing to cooperate, and floorboards shaking as Alice jumped. We eventually sat down to burnt lasagne at 11.50 p.m. Miranda and Roger were speechless, partly owing to the amount of alcohol they had consumed to survive the evening, but mainly because they could not believe what they had witnessed.

It was obvious to everyone who knew and loved us that I was not managing at home. Unbeknown to me, Miranda and Ian contacted my mother and sister, and summoned them to come to see me and insist that I should have Alice admitted to the unit full time. Without realising there was a strategy behind their two-day visit, I was looking forward to seeing them tremendously. In order to avoid disruption of our mornings and evenings, I suggested they stay at the local B&B, but I hoped that during the day we could have good times when we could visit Alice and I could share my anxieties with people I loved and trusted.

It was the most gruelling two days. My sister advised me, with the best of intentions, that I was handling the situation badly and that since Alice was obviously not making any progress I should insist that she be admitted full time. She also told me that I was being unfair to Ian, Beth and Jenny. I tried to defend my reasoning, repeating the consultant's advice that it was in Alice's best interests to remain at home and that I feared she would lose the positive thread she had clung on to if admitted against her will. I knew I was totally immersed in Alice's illness, but I was continually receiving her desperate letters:

> *I sometimes wonder whether I can manage another day and I know you must too. But I will if you will because without you I really am lost in a deep and incredibly dark hole . . . but Pinky is still there.*

Alice also held a deep-rooted conviction that we were all conspiring against her,

> *I really do wonder if at times people want to give up on*

62

*me. I don't want people to leave me alone fighting this but
I think that sometimes people just think 'leave her behind'.*

Alice understood the hell she was putting us through, as I
had seen from some of her letters, but those same letters
implied that she was determined that we could beat it. As
long as Alice believed that we were in some way making
progress, I had to support her. If the hospital insisted that
Alice be admitted, I would then respect their decision but I
wanted it to be the professionals' decision rather than mine.
I think my mother knew I was nearly at the end of my
tether but could understand that I had to be allowed to
judge the situation for myself.

Ian, however, put me under intolerable pressure, continually insisting that Alice be admitted as soon as possible. One
day I simply flipped and tried to get out of the moving car
on the way to the unit. Villagers enjoying a quiet evening
drink looked on with interest as a black car passed by with
a hysterical woman hanging out. Ian was shaken by the inci-
dent – I was desperate, and at my wits' end.

I found the weekly family therapy sessions extremely
helpful during this period. Although Alice never looked
forward to them, she was prepared to participate. Through
them she gave me an insight into some of her thoughts, even
though she would not confront her anorexia. I, too, could
express some of my emotions, though I didn't disclose the
full horror of what was happening at home. The professionals encouraged a 'collaborative' approach where
anything that needed to be said should be openly discussed
between us all. Alice loathed the idea of anyone talking
about her behind her back, but I felt inhibited by her presence.

I felt that if Alice had been suffering from a different kind of chronic illness, her progress, or lack of it, would have been totally in the hands of the professionals and I would not be open to so much free 'advice' from others outside, which exhausted and frustrated me. Perhaps this was the start of my story – I longed for someone to just listen to all my doubts and fears without comment, advice or analysis.

I hit a crisis point when David accepted an invitation from the consultant to attend a 'review meeting' in August. Since our divorce he had made very little effort to be responsible for his children either emotionally or financially, which had infuriated me. However, I always encouraged them to keep in contact with him and they visited him by choice about once a year. Although he was an absentee father, I didn't think this was the explanation for Alice's anorexia, and I always believed that he loved them all. But I had become increasingly frustrated that he had shown a lack of interest in Alice's rapid decline. As well as ignoring our phone calls, he had never responded to the unit, which had kept him informed of developments. Alice herself had commented that other children's fathers had flown in from abroad to visit their children in the unit, but her father obviously did not think she was ill enough to make the three-hour drive to visit her. He had always made me feel inferior, and I was very apprehensive at the prospect of a difficult meeting in his presence. The unit, therefore, offered us the option of two separate meetings, but Alice wanted us to meet together. It would be the first time in seven years that the three children and their parents were in the same room.

The unit wanted to address a number of problems at the meeting, including Alice's consistently low weight and her increased jumping and vomiting. The staff were also uncertain as to whether her behaviour was OCD-driven or anorexic-based. (They had suggested giving Alice medication during the previous few weeks but she had consistently refused to consider this option.)

By the time the big day arrived I had broken two phones and one vacuum cleaner and crashed my car into a tree, due to the frustration and anger of too many people telling me what I should do. And I had received a vitriolic letter from David condemning me on many issues since our divorce, for which he received just as vitriolic a response. Any chances of having a conciliatory meeting were blown.

Paramount in my mind was Alice's well-being, and, however difficult the situation was going to be, it must not harm her in any way.

In order to keep my composure during the appointment I decided to read from notes that Beth, Jenny and Ian all agreed beforehand were a fair reflection of life at home. They gave an honest account of Alice's jumping and vomiting, and, for the first time, I was prepared to disclose the full extent of her behaviour. Reluctantly, the three of them accepted that I would not be asking for Alice's admission. If I was going to betray Alice at the meeting, I was not prepared to ask for her admission at the same time.

The meeting, no doubt, was as difficult for David as for the rest of us, but all the children were pleased to see him. He was unsure how to react to Alice, who was a changed individual from the last time he'd seen her, and he asked me what he should do. I suggested that he give her a hug.

During the meeting David listened while the professionals and I gave our views on Alice's progress, or lack of it. His assessment was that it was apparent that Alice did not want to get better. I was angry because I felt that he had made no effort to encourage her otherwise, and so I was appalled when he was invited to attend the next meeting.

The meeting concluded that Alice would be put on one-to-one nursing care during her time at the unit, and that her refusal of medication would be assessed at the next meeting. Alice would continue to come home 'with a clear and detailed' plan, but it was agreed that if this was not successful Alice would need to be admitted. The final sentence of the review reiterated everything that the unit had been warning me for the last couple of months: that the illness was a marathon, 'The nature and severity of Alice's illness means that she is likely to remain ill for quite some time. Progress will be more in terms of her learning to control her illness and developing motivation to do so.'

I resorted to the sanctuary of my car, lit a cigarette and wept. I could not comprehend why the unit was so keen to involve Alice's father, who would simply drive away and reappear a month later. Inevitably, there was a scene between us in the car park. Although Alice was not present, our two eldest children were horrified to witness it. I eventually explained to David that if he were to be included in the programme he must be prepared to do some homework by either phoning or writing to Alice regularly.

We had a family therapy meeting scheduled for the beginning of the following week, but for the first time in Alice's treatment I did not feel able to participate. I could not manage the combination of an anorexic daughter and the complicated relationship of an estranged husband/father that the unit was asking me to handle. Unless David was prepared to participate in the day-to-day responsibility of Alice, why should he be included?

Alice's illness was exposing every possible weakness in our lives, and I was mortified.

Beth and Alice went to the meeting without me and discussed the complicated relationship they had with their father. Without my knowledge, Ian contacted the unit and tried to explain the enormous difficulties I was experiencing both with Alice and, emotionally, with her father. It resulted in another meeting early the following week with all the staff connected with Alice's care, as well as Alice and Beth. Ian, too, was asked to attend, but although I encouraged his presence he still could not be persuaded to come. At the meeting a number of issues were discussed, the first being 'whether Alice's mother is so overwhelmed or so manipulated by her daughter that she is unable to function as a parent and needs decisions made for her'. It was destroying to have the professionals imply that I was so incompetent. I replied that I was confident that this was not the case and that I was still capable of being a responsible mother.

As the meeting progressed it became apparent that perhaps there had not been sufficient communication between staff and home and it was agreed that we needed a tighter and more measured programme of combined goals, expectations and assessments of improvement. Weekly meetings with Alice, myself, nursing staff and the cognitive therapist would be arranged. Targets would be set and progress carefully monitored. If we continued to fall short of achieving these at home, but Alice was managing better at the unit, it would provide a strong argument for Alice being admitted full time. The consultant also advised Alice that if she continued to be 'stuck' and not moving forward with the programme, he would insist that he would be unable to help her unless she took medication. Her father received a letter explaining that he would not be invited to the next meeting after all, but he would still be encouraged to become involved in Alice's life.

Shortly after this I met the cognitive therapist who had been working with Alice. I knew Alice really enjoyed her times with him and he obviously knew and understood her. It was a relief to be in a meeting where there was some humour, and the three of us could openly discuss her behaviour. I couldn't comprehend the complexities of the routines that were controlling Alice but they now seemed to revolve around counting in sequences of six. With the help of the therapist Alice devised a plan whereby very slowly she would aim to reduce some of her rigmaroles. We knew the task she was undertaking was tremendously difficult and would require enormous commitment and encouragement to succeed. That night when I brought her home I felt better than I had for weeks, as I had a structure to work with. Alice, too, seemed excited and full of optimism.

Our first night was positive, Alice congratulated herself on missing out a fragment of everything and I was delighted that she went to bed pleased with herself. It was a joy to tuck her into her 'cotton wool bed' with a smile on her face rather than complete torment. But as the days went by I became more and more baffled by Alice's so-called victories, and I really couldn't see any improvements. One evening I asked her if I could write down each ritual and the number sequence behind it so that I could follow her routines. However, there were so many 'variations' of number six: (2×3) (6×1) (6×2) (4×3) $(3 + 3)$, and adaptations of jumping routines to match the numbers, and it went on and on. We met weekly with the cognitive therapist during this period and, much as we all wanted Alice to be winning, by the end of August 2001 I think Alice had accepted that we were beaten.

Soon afterwards I did not find it too difficult to hold up my hand and ask for Alice's full-time admission as soon as possible. I didn't feel I was betraying Alice any more; I felt that I had tried my best but that wasn't enough to get her better. I never spoke directly to her over this issue but one day she asked me to buy her some new pyjamas and I knew she had reached the same conclusion.

On a personal level, I had travelled through new depths of emotions. Never before had I experienced such feelings of loneliness, despair and fear, and any confidence I had left had dwindled as Alice's decline continued. I had spent more than two months engulfed by her jumping and her alien behaviour, and by the time she was admitted her weight gain was negligible even though her meal plan was enormous. Love was not enough to get Alice better; this was going to prove a huge learning curve. Alice gave me a clue when she wrote:

> *I hate the restrictions and anorexia hates it even more, but I need help with control.*

CHAPTER 5

Darkness and Light

So, in September 2001, we began the next stage of Alice's journey. Jenny came home to help me pack Alice's things for her stay as a full-time inpatient at the unit. She knew it was going to be a difficult day for us and her support was invaluable. Alice, too, was relieved to see her. At the unit we tried to make Alice's room look like home: flowers in a pot, photos on the wall, and I was given instructions to find some jolly posters. Jenny and I left Alice looking terrified, not angry. How on earth she was going to cope with all her routines in this new environment and discipline I could not imagine.

The unit very quickly put Alice on bed-rest and 24-hour one-to-one nursing care. She was devastated. All her 'treats' were removed: no 20-minute walks, no recreational activities of any kind, no watching television in the sitting room. She was allowed to participate in the unit's school lessons each day but otherwise she had to stay on her bed. Our Saturday outings were cancelled. And, finally, she succumbed to accepting medication.

I received suicidal phone calls from her, pleading with me to take her home, and more beseeching letters:

I feel as though I've cried all afternoon. I am so unhappy here and really think I could manage at home. Every time I try to make an effort to cut out something (i.e. break down my jumping) they take more away from me . . . I don't know how I can fight all my battles when they take more and more away from me. I don't know how to stay positive. I just wish one thing would go 'for me' rather than 'against me'. It's awful – Pinky is so exhausted and I honestly wonder how long she can last.

But however desperate she was, I knew coming home was not the answer. I visited her each day and although she was then at an all-time low – extremely withdrawn and totally consumed by her own mental torment – small things reassured me that Alice was receiving better care than I could provide for her at home: the unit provided a soft fleecy type of mattress for her to sleep on, to protect her thin body from bedsores, and one day she told me grudgingly that a night nurse had smothered her hands completely with hand cream, wrapped them up in a pair of socks and assured her that in the morning they would look much better.

We were back to long weekends at the unit with Alice, and it was harder than ever to find some kind of activity that would help to pass the time. Alice was totally immersed in her world of jumping and anorexia. Although I was with her when the disaster of 11 September 2001 was reported on the television in the unit, it wasn't until a year later when the images were repeated that I realised how little she had taken in at the time. She watched the repeat of the disaster with complete disbelief as the horrors unfolded and said that she had never seen any of it before. It was a frightening revelation for both of us.

Although all responsibilities for Alice's day-to-day care were in the hands of the unit, I felt that I could still provide emotional support. My visits were a relief for Alice, the one-to-one nursing care was less obvious and she could have some privacy. I tried to take in something each day that would amuse her, if only for a tiny time: stickers, flowers, bubbles, music and a copy of *Alice in Wonderland*, which I hoped might capture her imagination. I left notes under her pillow each night. (I remembered my GP saying months before that he had a patient who had suffered from anorexia for years, and one day a piece of music had provided the answer for her). One day I took in a couple of posters: one of flags of the world, which I thought she could memorise during the long hours on bed-rest, and the other a world map. Initially, Alice was angry: 'For goodness sake, Mum, I'm fifteen!' The flags never made it to the wall but in the weeks to follow the world map did seem to have an impact. Alice and her fellow inmates had happy times plotting and marking their adventures ahead. Who knows, perhaps Alice was just being polite, or perhaps the map did indeed give her some incentive to aim for the future.

By this time it was clear that Alice would not now be attending school for quite a considerable time. She had missed the last month of year ten but had managed to complete most of the curriculum for that year.

Alice's school and the unit had been communicating about her education and progress during her admission, and by September it was apparent that this would have to continue, as Alice would not be returning to school in the foreseeable future. Fortunately the unit was blessed with an exceptional teacher who offered to visit the school with Alice and me to discuss Alice's education.

Alice inevitably set herself extremely high standards and was adamant that she would continue with all her chosen subjects in spite of my suggestions that she drop some of them. Although I may once have been an ambitious parent, Alice's educational merits now seemed trivial compared to her health. However, she began the year of her GCSE examinations under one-to-one nursing care and with a determination that I could only admire.

I arranged a second appointment for Ian and me with the headmaster of the boarding school that we had liked during our visit in the early spring. Education was the one aspect of life where Alice showed any interest, and the prospect of studying for her A levels at this school did seem to provide some kind of incentive for her. Since the age of 14 she had set her heart on studying medicine, and, though I really couldn't see any possible likelihood of her being well enough to achieve her goal, I certainly was not going to destroy her dreams. The headmaster asked how Alice was progressing and I explained that she was in hospital suffering from anorexia and that I had no idea how she would be by the following September, but that I would like her to join the school if she were well enough. He wished her well and said that the school would have to assess Alice closer to the time, but should she join the school they would do everything possible to accommodate her needs. I left feeling sad; two years earlier any school would have been lucky to have Alice and now I was asking for help.

I had continued to attend the parents' meetings at the unit throughout this period and looked forward to the two-weekly sessions. I formed new friendships and sometimes among all the horror stories we could laugh as we exchanged ghastly experiences. Up to this point I really had very little to contribute, but it was fascinating listening to others. There were parents who were pleased with their child's progress, parents who were experiencing their child's second or third admission, parents who were preparing for their child's discharge and parents whose child had been discharged. Although Alice's discharge seemed an eternity away, I listened avidly to these parents. For once I was ahead of the game and was receiving information before encountering the problem. I formed a particular friendship with a mother whose daughter was experiencing her first admission to this hospital but had endured two other admissions, one in a psychiatric ward of a general hospital and one in another adolescent eating disorders unit. She was a lovely lady, quiet but wise. She had spent the past three years driving around England and finally moving house in order to be close to her daughter. If I thought I had problems, she'd had worse.

Within a month as a full-time inpatient Alice had gained control of her jumping. Qualified, confident professionals could impose on Alice a discipline that I never could. The medication obviously had a large part to play, not for the anorexia but for the OCD. I later asked Alice why she had been so ardently resistant to taking medication and was amazed that her answer was 'because it might make me better'. I had thought it was because of the fear of unknown calories. When asked by the family therapist what explanation I could give for Alice's progress, my views were: exceptional professional care, medication and also the fact that by the time Alice was admitted we were at rock bottom. Behind these criteria was a deep belief that Alice did indeed want to get out of this hell.

By October 2001 we had turned a corner. Alice was beginning to follow the programme and I took it as an opportunity to return to basics and put into play everything that I had learnt during the past year.

I practised keeping to the rules the unit had established during family meals at the unit. I mastered the scales, learnt the different cutlery, plates and glasses that Alice required and, most importantly, I learnt not to run late. If everything was prepared correctly first time, we did not have too many difficulties. If something was wrong − perhaps I put the wrong spoon on the tray or her glass of water was not filled to the correct level − Alice would become agitated. I also knew I must not give her any reason that might result in my having to leave the room, thus giving her the opportunity to jump or to hide her food. I had never been an organised person, but I realised that when Alice came home I was going to have to become far more efficient in my shopping and meal preparation than I had ever been before so that I would not be out-manoeuvred by Alice's illness.

The Saturdays at the unit became less of a battle. One afternoon Alice sat on the sofa plaiting a nurse's long hair and allowed me to try to plait hers for over an hour. It was the first time for more than three months that, without argument, she had sat quietly for one and a half hours. I knew we must maintain this when she came home.

When I joined her in the patients' dining room while she ate her snack in the afternoon, I began to appreciate the extraordinary amount of food that Alice was expected to eat each day. I watched my child, who had a complete terror of food, eat more than any 'ordinary' person would eat each day. Her snack at teatime was three Jaffa cakes, an apple and a large glass of juice. Only a couple of hours before, she had eaten a large lunch and had been instructed to sit quietly in between meals. An enormous supper was to follow shortly. What a nightmare for her.

Until now Alice had been reluctant to see her friends, though she had been writing to them and receiving their letters over the previous weeks. Her dear friend Nuala had been wonderfully loyal towards Alice during the months before her admission and I kept in touch with her regularly. She was looking forward to seeing Alice again and so I suggested to Alice that it might be a good idea if I brought Nuala into the unit one afternoon. In spite of Alice's anxiety about her best friend seeing her in such an environment, I brought Nuala in, having explained to her all about the unit first. The pair had a happy time and agreed that they would meet up again soon. It was a glimpse of normality to see the two teenagers gossiping. Nuala's contribution was exceptional; she became involved in the programme as much as any of us, she visited Alice often, measured food for family meals at the unit, accompanied Alice on her walks and together we learnt the regimes of Alice's new life.

While Alice was safe in the unit and apparently making progress, Beth and Jenny pointed out that perhaps it was time for Ian to have some more of my time. It was a fair suggestion but I didn't in any way want to penalise Alice for doing well. I plucked up the courage to tell Alice that I would not be visiting her on Sundays – she accepted it surprisingly well, and was pleased to think that I would be having a good time.

However, a rift was widening between Alice and Jenny. Jenny had understandably found the past months painful and felt that I had become totally preoccupied with Alice (though she had been the focus of my energies while she struggled with A levels only the previous year). Jenny was also very firm in her manner towards Alice's eating habits and would not tolerate any unnecessary excuses, and Alice found this difficult.

Ian, however, was excited at the prospect of an entire Sunday with me to himself, as he had found the past few months extremely lonely. And so for our first Sunday of independence we drove to the coast, then just walked and talked. We had a relaxing pub lunch and it was heaven to do normal things again.

Nuala was brilliant, as usual, and happily agreed to visit Alice in the unit on Sundays and encouraged other friends to join them.

Alice continued to improve at the unit. Her weight began to increase, and one evening she completed the entire shower routine without a jump. Her humour also began to return. It was time for her to come home for a day and see if we could manage.

Both of us were extremely nervous. Alice had to face the ultimate test of controlling her rigmaroles in the environment where they had been most dominant. With the family therapist's help we had agreed on a plan for the day: a quiet morning, lunch at home, an outing in the afternoon and then back to the unit for supper. I prepared everything by the book, and a previous conversation with the staff and Alice at the unit confirmed what I had really always known: 'Healthy Eating' cottage cheese was not acceptable.

As I drove in to collect Alice I felt sick with apprehension. Remarkably, she got into the car and sat quietly all the way home. She got out of the car, walked into the house and smiled. She was going to manage. We had a good morning, a 20-minute walk before lunch, lunch at the table set out as it would be in the unit, one hour quiet time after it and then into the town for a couple of hours. When I returned Alice to the unit that afternoon we were both over the moon. We had completed a day with no 'ifs' or 'buts'. It was the most momentous day for me.

During the following month our times at home increased until Alice was spending entire weekends at home. However, our fridge by now had very definite divisions between Ian's and my food and Alice's food, as Alice could not bring herself to touch a pack of butter and she was permanently concerned that her ingredients had in some way been contaminated by a rogue calorie. I was particularly nervous preparing her suppers. The food in the unit nick-named 'cooked chill' was pretty unappetising and I hoped that home-cooked food would in some way be an improvement. The unit provided me with a meal plan that detailed everything Alice would be expected to eat throughout the day, but supper was the most ambiguous because it was described in weight rather than ingredients (for example, 200g 'main dish', 210g creamed potatoes). Alice was still eating a considerable amount of food and when I served her first supper of baked fish I realised that it was really an impossible amount of fish for anyone to eat.

I had to come up with another plan and decided on a basic tomato sauce to accompany the fish. I developed endless variations of tomato sauce, adding different vegetables, herbs and spices and I became very efficient at freezing small batches, which could accompany chicken and prawns. I followed the meal plan religiously as her stays at home extended. It was tempting to cheat and add extra oil to the sauce but I decided against it. Alice had to build up her trust in me and if she ever found out that her meals were not 'safe' it would cause irreparable damage. Also, in the long term Alice had to learn what she had to eat to stay well, and realistically I didn't think extra oil would be on her menu. The table was set, the food was cooked at the correct time, and I became more confident and quicker at preparing her meals. However, they continued to take up a sizeable part of each day – it took Alice about an hour to eat each meal and we maintained the quiet hour after each – but we were managing at last.

The unit was delighted with Alice's improvement. One-to-one nursing care was removed and she was 'promoted' to another bedroom along the corridor rather than having the room directly opposite the nurse's office. She progressed from being one of the least positive patients in the unit to a 'positive' patient, and sometimes I would walk in and hear laughter among her and her friends down the corridor. It was wonderful.

One evening Alice and I went out for supper with a fellow patient from the unit and her mother. It was a tremendously successful exercise; the children went shopping on their own first and we arranged to meet them at a 'friendly eating' restaurant at 6.30 p.m. The girls encouraged each other and it was a great relief to share the anxiety of our first meal out with another parent experiencing the same problems. On another evening the unit decided that Alice was well enough to join an outing to the cinema. She succeeded in keeping still during the film, and the praise she received from both patients and staff was heart-warming.

Slowly Alice began to socialise outside of the unit with Nuala and her other friends, meeting them for Saturday afternoon shopping excursions. Bonfire Night was the first night out when she wouldn't know exactly who she might bump into, but she was excited at the prospect of being back in the mainstream of life again. I dreaded some wise guy saying something that would knock her off course, and we discussed how she would react to any difficult comments. I am sure Alice spent considerable time mentally preparing herself for the hurdles that lay ahead.

In early November the unit encouraged her to attempt one day at school. Alice had kept up with her schoolwork as much as possible, with the encouragement of the teacher in the unit and the invaluable support of the science teacher from her school, who visited her a couple of times while she was there.

Alice and I planned her school day. We arranged that I would drive her to school rather than her taking the school bus and that Nuala would meet us at the school gate. With mixed emotions and some excitement, we set off. My admiration for Alice was enormous and as I watched the pair of them walking away I wished I could put her in a sandwich board that read 'I'm fragile – please handle with extreme care'. This was 'normality' – how would she manage, and how would people manage her? I would meet Alice at lunchtime so that she could eat her lunch in the car – she was still taking about an hour to eat – and she would return with Nuala for afternoon school. I hoped to avoid allowing Alice the chance of disappearing to the loo after lunch.

The day went well and I met Alice at the end of the day. She was happy but totally exhausted, and by the time we had driven the 20 minutes home she was asleep in the car.

Throughout the next month Alice increased her time at home until she was spending Thursdays, Fridays and Mondays at school, including the weekend in between at home, and then she stayed at the unit on Tuesdays and Wednesdays. It was a time when we both appreciated that we had to build up our confidence and trust in each other if we were going to survive without the day-to-day support of the unit. Alice had huge mood swings: she was either as high as a kite or exhausted; sometimes she was 15, sometimes she was eight and sometimes she was a little old lady.

On 3 December 2001 Alice was discharged from the unit, with weekly outpatient appointments to be arranged. Although she was still very thin, her weight was stable within her target range. She was attending school three days a week, and spending weekends at home where we were managing her meals and exercising, though it was tremendously time-consuming. We maintained the quiet hour after each meal if she was not at school or with her friends. I rarely let her out of my sight: I continued to chat to her upstairs while she was in the bath or getting ready for bed. She wanted the company and it prevented the opportunity for any jumping routines to return. Her mood was bright and enthusiastic.

Alice struggled with her body image but she was looking forward to being at home and at school full time and leading one life rather than a split one. It wasn't until she was discharged from the hospital that I fully realised the problems she had encountered with her body image – feeling that she was larger than she was and the genuine depth of discomfort and fear that an increase of 0.5kg presented to her. She was equally uncomfortable in or out of her clothes. She had discussed these issues with Sarah as well as during psycho-education sessions at the unit.

Alice had experienced the worst six months of her life during her time in hospital. She had built remarkable friendships with some of her fellow patients – one boy and eight girls. The letters and cards she received amazed me; they were all so encouraging and I still cannot begin to understand how some of the children could write such inspiring letters of well-being wishes but were unable to take the risk of attempting to overcome anorexia for themselves. How could we possibly thank enough those staff who had reached out and found the Alice of happier times and given us something to build on?

I reread the final sentence of her discharge notes several times: 'It has been a great pleasure working with Alice and seeing her through so well. We should, however, not be surprised if there are further difficulties that need some attention.'

Both she and I were hugely nervous on shutting the door on what had been our sanctuary during the past six months.

CHAPTER 6

After the Honeymoon

When Alice left the unit phrases from parents whose children had been discharged kept going round in my head: 'it's like having a baby again'; 'when the honeymoon period is over'; 'it's difficult to know which is the teenage daughter and which is the anorexic daughter'; 'never miss a meal', and so on. These gave me a clue that we were far from the finishing post. As well as the problems Alice had with food and her body image, she had to contend with her brain telling her that if she sat down for very long she was being lazy. She still had a small jumping routine each time she went to the loo, and always carefully handwashed, rinsed and re-rinsed all plates, glasses, knives and forks before she felt they were safe to use. Also, she had not been left on her own at any time, either at the hospital or at home, for well over six months, and had to overcome a fear of being left alone for even the shortest period.

While Alice had been ill for the past two years, her friends had grown into assured and confident 16-year-olds. One day she admitted that it was difficult to find anything in common with her friends any more; they chatted about boys, going clubbing, and eating pizzas, and all she really wanted to talk about was the number of calories in her sandwich.

Because she couldn't apply the word 'anorexia' to herself, she adopted a somewhat madcap persona. Perhaps the easiest disguise for her was to come across to her friends as a bit bonkers because that was what was expected of her. Although sometimes she was extremely amusing, there were other times when she was quite embarrassing and I wondered where it would all lead. Ian's daughter Olivia, who by now was something of a celebrity on the local radio station, and her boyfriend Kier were wonderful – they, too, could have mad moments and Alice built up a marvellous friendship with the pair of them. She also decided to go for a change of image. She had her long hair cut into a shorter, 'funkier' style and updated her wardrobe. Clothes sizes, however, were a delicate issue, as Alice's inclination was always towards size 6 rather than size 8. I wanted her to feel happy and confident in what she wore but hoped to encourage her away from such tiny sizes.

Her mood swings were enormous but the one constant was that at the end of every day she was utterly exhausted from her efforts of managing another 'normal' day. To make the school day flow smoothly for Alice, I made sure that the teachers knew she was still very fragile and the science teacher continued to support Alice as before. Nuala followed our plans to the letter every day and Alice successfully completed the Christmas term.

To some extent normality returned to the house. Ian came for supper each night, though Alice ate earlier, as she wanted to get her meals over and done with, and if they were weighed and prepared correctly she ate them. We continued with the quiet hour after supper. I knew Alice had a tendency to 'get stuck' with her rigmaroles if she was left on her own while she got ready for bed so I continued to chat to her upstairs while she had her bath and prepared for bed. She had changed to daily disposable contact lenses, which resolved the problems she had experienced before. As time went on we agreed on ways by which she could attempt to reduce some of her rituals.

The next major hurdle was Christmas itself. During the parents' meetings we had already discussed the difficulties that birthdays and other celebrations brought with them; Alice still could not sit at a table with anything as obviously dangerous as butter or cream on it, and she couldn't even get food out of the fridge if it was anywhere near such a threat. However, Miranda and her family invited us to spend Christmas with them and Alice agreed that this was a good plan; we would cook and weigh her meal at home, safely away from the turkey and roast potatoes, and microwave it at Miranda's. She agreed to have her main meal at lunchtime, which was going to be later than the usual 12.30 p.m., and would therefore eat her afternoon snack in the morning. She wanted us all to have a good Christmas and was willing to adapt so that we could.

For the first time in a very long time Alice had fun participating in the preparations for a celebration. She enjoyed choosing presents for her friends, wrapping them up and hoping that they would give pleasure, and we had a very happy Christmas.

We continued to have weekly appointments at the unit, when Alice's weight was monitored and she had the oppor-tunity to talk and plan with Sarah, the nurse who had known Alice during her inpatient treatment. We also had monthly review meetings and monthly appointments with the family therapist, but Alice found it increasingly difficult to return to the unit. As the weeks went by her friends were discharged and she found herself in alien territory worrying about how her weight compared with the new patients. She preferred to go the unit looking rather grim, wearing old clothes and no make-up. However, her times with Sarah were always constructive and, behind closed doors, no doubt she could converse with someone who understood and identified with the problems she was experiencing. I was immensely grateful for all the expertise that Sarah gave, but their conversations were private and, apart from changes in meal plans, which reflected weight gain or loss, I didn't know too much of what was said.

I was thrilled when Alice decided to celebrate New Year by having a party for friends. Ian and I left them to it, feeling rather nervous. We returned home at 1.00 a.m. to find an immaculate house and Alice somewhat blotto. My reaction was delight – how extraordinary to come home and find a drunk daughter, and be pleased!

By the end of the Christmas holidays Alice had lost a little weight but managed to keep just within her target range. Before she was discharged she had agreed on a weight zone variance of 2kg. Sarah advised us that I should resume making Alice's sandwiches – it was the only part of her food that was not weighed and Alice was obviously not quite managing to fill her sandwich sufficiently. Alice was still 'experiencing herself as fat and could find it very easy to start missing food', the consultant wrote, and it was agreed that for the time being She needed to keep a tight grip on her anorexic control as any undue flexibility would increase the risk of her relapsing. I mentioned to Sarah that I was having big problems in finding ways to reassure Alice about her body image. Sarah sympathised but said that while she had been a qualified specialist nurse for a long time, there was no obvious answer that she could give me.

So the spring term began, and rather than having lunch with me in the car as before, Alice began to have it with Nuala and other friends in a classroom. This was progress but Alice still felt unable to cope with the school canteen.

One blot on the horizon was the school ski trip that we had booked over a year previously. Alice was excited about it, especially when I gave her some ski socks and goggles for Christmas. By January, however, it was obvious that she would not be able to manage a week away from the structured routine that we had developed. I dreaded telling her that she would not be able to cope with the rigours of a ski trip, but one evening I tackled the subject. Although extremely disappointed, Alice reluctantly accepted that she would not be able to go.

Ian was suffering his own personal problems, too. His youngest daughter Heidi lived close by, but we had seen less and less of her since Alice had been admitted to hospital, and Ian missed her. He offered to take the four of us to Le Touquet during the half-term that Alice should have spent skiing. It was a generous and wonderful idea, and we were all excited.

We booked a two-night stay in a hotel. As it was off-season the hotel restaurant was closed, so we would have to find our meals ourselves. Alice discussed with Sarah during her weekly appointment how to approach the vagueness of the meals that lay ahead. We decided to take as many basic ingredients as possible with us in the car so that we could cover breakfast and lunch with the scales, but supper was going to be a wild card. Alice accepted that supper was going to be a risk but was confident that we would be able to find a simple fish dish that she would be prepared to eat in the evening in a restaurant and would be guided by me as to how much she should eat.

We had a happy two days, though the evening meals were extremely difficult, mainly because the service was slow, and during the time before the meal arrived Alice became increasingly quiet and anxious.

When we left Le Touquet we planned to take the girls to City Europe before catching the shuttle home in time for supper. As Heidi had her sixth-form ball coming up, and Alice had her school prom in May, it seemed like the ideal opportunity for the two of them to find the perfect dress. Heidi eventually found one that looked wonderful, but Alice had still not found the dress of her dreams. It wasn't until we passed the Disney Store that Alice's eyes lit up. We came home with a Disney *Monster's Inc.* outfit for her prom.

Nevertheless, we had covered new ground. Although Alice had lost weight during our three-day trip away, the trip had been a success. Ian had a lovely time with Heidi, and Alice and Heidi had both enjoyed themselves a great deal. I had loved the change of routine but realised that Alice was still extremely limited by her illness and that the very structured routine of home was still essential. With Sarah's help Alice regained her lost weight during the next few weeks.

At the review meeting in mid-March 2002 the team agreed that Alice was continuing to do very well: her weight was in the target range, she was socialising and her progress was all the more impressive because she continued to 'suffer from strong anorexic thoughts and feelings'. I was delighted and told Alice how extremely proud of her I was. However, I found Alice's friendships with fellow patients from the unit a difficult matter to manage; I didn't know whether to encourage them or suggest that she leave them behind in her attempts to move on to 'normality'. She received several letters and phone calls, but quickly lost touch with others who had been great friends. Was she in contact with the children who were moving forward, or the ones who were struggling? It was difficult to know. One weekend I agreed that a friend from the unit could come and stay for a night. Her mother and I were confident that it would be a successful stay. The two children were on similar meal plans and we were both of the opinion that although it wasn't easy, we were moving forward rather than back. It proved a mistake; the two girls hadn't seen each other for a while and although they got on well together it was obvious from the first moment that they were eyeing each other up to see who was thinnest.

On the plus side, Alice was expanding on the 'alternatives' to her meal plan. Although she continued to spend hours in Tesco looking at calories and the fat content of different items, one day we came home with a Crunchie chocolate bar rather than a yogurt, which she assured me was the equivalent in calories. I was ecstatic. Surely this was progress if Alice was eating chocolate?

The Easter holiday arrived and I tried to make sure that we had a plan for each day. We hadn't seen my mother or sister since the unfortunate weekend in September and Alice seemed happy with the idea that they should come and stay for Easter. We had a happy time but inevitably with ten ordinary people in the house, a considerable amount of time was spent sitting, eating and chatting.

It was difficult keeping such a close eye on Alice. All her meals were weighed and cooked as usual, but I was somewhat distracted by other home activities, and I didn't really notice that she had taken to eating her yogurt standing by the radiator rather than sitting at the table as usual. The one-hour quiet times after meals were sometimes interrupted, though I continued to chat to her while she was in the bath and always made sure that she was safely tucked up in bed at the end of each day.

Alice began to look a little thinner and became quieter. The speed at which she began to lose ground took my breath away. We saw Sarah each week and she changed the meal plan because Alice was losing weight, but Alice seemed to be eating her meals – I couldn't understand where we were going wrong. After three weeks Alice finally admitted that she was being sick again. Sarah warned Alice that within another couple of weeks of such obvious weight loss we would be back at the starting post. I drove home terrified – could Alice turn it around?

That night I wrote out a list of where I thought we'd gone wrong:

- Alice's review meeting had backfired. She found it difficult to be 'a good anorexic'.

- It was a mistake to have a friend from the unit to stay. They competed.

- The stress of schoolwork.

- I didn't pay sufficient attention to her calorie conversions and equivalents.

- During the quiet hour she sometimes slipped upstairs.

- Boredom during the holidays.

- Too much food and chatting over Easter meant that Alice was excluded.

- Late to bed and tiredness.

At the end I wrote 'I must return to basics.' I tightened up on everything. Alice and I sat together quietly during every meal and the one hour of quiet time afterwards. I also insisted that she return to the table for her yogurt. I accompanied her every time she went upstairs. Jenny and I sat down with a calculator and worked out the calorie content of the equivalents that Alice had been experimenting with. It quickly became obvious that she had reduced her meal plan significantly. I told Alice the choice was hers: she could either go back down the slippery slope or I would do everything possible to help her climb her way back. I watched and waited for the dreaded jumping to return.

Miraculously, Alice began to claw back her weight over the next month, during which time I made every effort to point out what she was gaining by the enormous effort she had put into the past few months: friends, school and a life that she was battling for, and, in so many ways, achieving. I have no doubt that if Alice had instead chosen to pursue the anorexic route nothing, I could have done could have dissuaded her.

Alice was 16 in the May of 2002, and we prepared for her final term at school. There were no changes to our approach the previous term except that I noticed that she was putting on some make-up during our drive to school. However, her 'wobble' over the Easter holiday had left its scars on me. My hitherto growing confidence had completely evaporated. I had made mistakes: I had been too easily persuaded to see progress when in fact I should have heard alarm bells; I had known anorexia was always breathing down Alice's neck but had not anticipated the speed of its tentacles.

Although we were back to as tight a regime as ever, I tried to take the emphasis away from meals. I didn't push her towards new ingredients, but kept her meals simple and safe, so that they could be approached with minimum anxiety. I focused on encouraging her to embrace life and find out that it could actually be fun, but I had to balance this with ensuring that she didn't get overtired or bored, as this would cause the problems to return. It was obvious that days with nothing planned were daunting for Alice, though she was reluctant to implement activities for herself and required some persuasion to pick up the phone and initiate any arrangements. If I saw a gap in my diary for a couple of days, we would formulate a plan to fill it, and I continued to encourage Alice to feel that she was making progress even though she had experienced her most negative period since her discharge.

At Sarah's suggestion Alice found herself a part-time job; it was at a restaurant quite close to home, where she would work on Sundays from 11.00 a.m. until 5.00 p.m. To begin with I was rather apprehensive that the combination of schoolwork, her new social life and working at the restaurant would prove too much for her, but she was excited at the prospect of earning some money and insisted that she would be able to manage. I pointed out also that she was going to be in close proximity to all the foods that she endeavoured to keep as far away from as possible. We formulated a plan as to how she would manage her meals during the six-hour period. We decided that she would have to have her breakfast and lunch before she left, so our 'restful' Sundays started with breakfast at 7.00 a.m. and lunch at 10.15 a.m.!

It was wonderful advice from Sarah. Alice managed all that was asked of her. In a new environment she learnt to pour cream and wipe and wash sticky plates and tables and this did her ego a tremendous amount of good. She was delighted with her progress and, of course, her pay packets.

Soon after, Sarah left the unit on maternity leave and handed over Alice's care to Gina. The changeover was handled with expertise and Alice was once again placed in the care of someone she could confide in and relate to.

As the exams loomed Nuala and Alice decided to meet up for revision sessions, which provided a further opportunity for Alice to expand her horizons. Some evenings she would take her scales and supper to Nuala's house (baked potato and baked beans were an easy menu to follow) and after a few weeks Alice spent the night away. Nuala was as consistent as ever, even missing her weekend sleep-in to join Alice at breakfast time.

Alice continued to pursue her interest in the boarding school that she had visited before the impact of her illness, and asked if she could return and reassure herself that the school was as she remembered it. This time we met the staff who would be directly responsible for her academic and pastoral care. We drove home with Alice confident that this was the school she was aiming for. I had enormous doubts, but thought that perhaps it would be a possibility on a 'day' basis rather than boarding, at least initially, and advised the school accordingly.

Then there was the prom dress. Alice decided that perhaps the monster outfit wasn't quite the thing, but it became a big issue and I felt that Alice was planning some kind of metamorphosis at the prom. She wanted to make an impression; she wanted her friends to see her as an attractive 16-year-old and not the Alice of the previous two years. We found the dress of her dreams and she did in fact look wonderful. I could have bust a gut with pride. My confidence began to grow. Alice had proved that she meant to keep moving on.

She completed all her GCSEs. With the arrival of the summer holidays we were still on as tight a regime as ever, as far as food and the scales were concerned, but we were managing and leading a normal life – on the surface at least. Sometimes I think Alice became frustrated with her lack of progress, but Gina and I would point out to her just how much progress she had already made. Gradually we made small adaptations to our routine. Instead of me following Alice every time she went upstairs, which must have been irritating, we began to sing to each other. We both knew she couldn't be sick while she was in full voice. If a friend of mine was visiting during a meal, Alice offered to eat her meal unaccompanied. I'd pop in to check she was OK and she knew that if there were any problems I would join her. It was a risk, but I felt that she needed the opportunity to prove that she could be trusted again. She had also taken to having a shower unaccompanied. Her hands were looking better and, without my really realising it, I wasn't putting hand cream on them every night before she went to sleep.

We kept our routines and I had a constant supply of drinks and snack bars in the car so that there would be no excuse for missing out on a meal. Sometimes, when we were at home, Alice would act strangely, opening and shutting cupboards, reaching for a glass and then not taking one. It was her way of telling me that I should have reminded her to have a snack. She explained that she felt greedy if the suggestion of food came from her rather than me. My role was to remove this pressure from her.

Our close friends continued to be understanding and they encouraged Alice and us all back into their lives. I asked them not to make any comments as to 'how well' she looked, which I knew she would interpret only in kilograms. Slowly we began to reclaim a social life and Alice came with us, adapting meals so that she would have the security of eating her own food.

Jenny came home for her summer vacation this time. She had another long summer of working in the celery fields to finance her way through her final year at university, and it gradually came to light how much she had resented my suggestion that she spend the previous summer with her boyfriend and how little I had seen her during the past year. I realised that I hadn't been back to London since her first day at university, so I hadn't seen the flat where she lived or met any of her new friends. We had some serious catching up to do.

The only time we all met up was when Beth and Jenny came home for weekends, and it took a while for everyone to adjust to each other. I had to explain to the girls the changes that had occurred since their last visit; for example, Alice was allowed to measure her own supper and prepare her own sandwich with one of us watching. But it was good for me to have a different opinion, and Jenny was excellent at pointing out areas that I had let slip. Without realising it, Ian and I had swapped roles over the past few months. He and Alice joked at my 'nagging'. He became the good guy and I was the baddie; everyone knew it was well-intentioned but looking back now I can see that I did become the disciplinarian. I found it easier to put myself in that role rather than having others tell me what I should be doing, and Alice appreciated my consistency.

Fifteen months had passed since our disastrous family holiday in the South of France and we were about to embark on a repeat exercise. We adopted a different game plan this time. Alice would stay for the full two weeks, and assorted children and friends would join us throughout the holiday. I was confident that we could make the holiday work this time.

However, Nuala arrived feeling unwell and had to spend a quiet week in the shade unable to participate. It was ghastly for her and, unfortunately, had repercussions on Alice. She found it increasingly difficult to eat her meals while her friend ate next to nothing, and the days seemed dreadfully long lazing around the pool. I was not surprised when the scales confirmed a loss of weight, but this time we did not have the unit to help us.

Alice admitted that she was having problems staving off the vomiting and I suggested that we would have to return to the familiar rigid routine. Amazingly, she was grateful.

We shared the second week with the same great friends who had shared the disastrous holiday with us the year before, but they were game to try another. We had a hysterical time; everything that could go wrong, went wrong, from a pneumatic drill banging away all day in our drive to a diver arriving one lunchtime dressed in his scuba gear to unblock the pool. But Alice won her battle.

At our review meeting shortly after our return it was agreed that Alice was continuing to make good progress, though 'Alice does continue to have strong anorexic thoughts and feelings. This means that the only way that she has been able to make her great strides forward has been by having very definite routines.' So it was decided that the routines should continue.

We planned the rest of the summer holidays so that Alice had some kind of activity to wake up to each morning. Her waitressing job continued and even increased to include a few evenings.

Although it was monotonous, Alice showed no desire to extend her menu so we continued with her familiar foods. Our singing sessions began to disappear and Alice gradually became responsible for herself after meals. Often she would nip upstairs shortly after a meal, and I found it extremely difficult not to follow her or ask her if everything was all right. Ian repeatedly pointed out to me that I must allow Alice this opportunity of independence.

For the first time in over two years Alice was looking well. The French sun had removed the translucent white of her skin, her eyes were bright and her face expressed happiness rather than torment. She was extremely thin but not appalling to the eye. She continued her weekly appointments with Gina during the summer and we enjoyed a period of Alice maintaining her weight in the middle of her target zone. Our sessions with the family therapist were becoming less frequent, though I still found them invaluable. It was during one of these appointments that Alice announced that she knew she would be unable to manage boarding school in September 2002 and accepted that at first she would start her new school as a day-girl. I was relieved that she had come to this decision on her own.

In earlier years Alice had gone on holiday to Cornwall with Nuala, her mum and friends of their family, and they

were keen for her to rejoin them this year. It was an opportunity for Alice to take another risk. I could send her off
with a list of instructions, scales and ingredients, but it would
be her responsibility to manage it all. I needed Gina to help
us devise a plan. The only measure I could relate to was the
scales, and Alice had to agree to being weighed at intervals
during her time away. However, if Alice chose to drink an
excessive amount of water before the weighing sessions, she
could beat the scales, and I would not be there to notice.

As it transpired, Alice returned home ten days later
having had a wonderful time and looking exceptionally
well. Amid all the stories of fun on the beach, sailing and
teenage banter, she revealed that had put a word to her
illness for the first time. During an evening of family games
everyone was asked to disclose their worst experiences of
that year. Alice knew she was in the company of friends who
knew, so it would come as no surprise, but she did admit that
she had been in hospital for six months suffering from
'anorexia'. And, most importantly, Alice had proved that she
could survive when left to her own devices.

The GCSE results came out the day after her return.
Alice had already achieved everything beyond my wildest
dreams for that year and I could hope for nothing more, but
when we received her results I realised that the determination that had done so much to harm her in the past had
produced remarkable results.

As the holidays came to a close we began to formulate a
plan for her new school life. An important part of the
strategy for Alice was that her peers should not know what
had gone on before, as she was bitterly ashamed of her
illness. She could take her lunch and snack bars and no one
would be the wiser. It seemed possible, until we received a

letter from the school giving the itinerary for the 'induction days'. Day pupils as well as boarders would be expected to stay overnight to enjoy a ceilidh on the first evening and a picnic outing on the second day.

I was delighted that the first thing that came to Alice's mind was excitement rather than apprehension, but it was a big hurdle to leap. One morning she announced that she would like to join the school as a weekly boarder rather than on a daily basis. If she was going to manage 48 hours, why not bite the bullet and become a boarder? I was staggered; Ian, to give him his due, had always believed Alice would achieve her goal.

I knew Alice would relish the life of a boarder. The days were structured, there would be very little time for any loneliness or boredom and she would love the camaraderie of her fellow students. She was thrilled when Gina encouraged her with the plan. We all knew Alice was frustrated by her lack of progress concerning meals but I had always envisaged a very gradual removal of the stipulations that had governed her eating habits until now.

A few days later Alice said that she wanted Ian and me to understand that boarding did not mean that this was the end of her eating disorder and we should not presume that it would be easy. I welcomed her acceptance of the problems ahead and knew my role was to make the transition as feasible as possible for her. It seemed monumental; Alice had spent the past 18 months knowing that all her meals were specially weighed and prepared, and now this support was going to be removed within the next two weeks.

I phoned the school explaining that there had been another change of plan and that Alice hoped to join as a weekly boarder. I was hugely encouraged when the head of catering suggested that she should meet Alice personally. We looked at the school menu and realised very quickly that it would be an impossible transition for Alice to make. Together we devised a plan of simple meals that could be provided without too much effort for the kitchen staff or embarrassment for Alice. Although every meal had been weighed down to the last exact gramme, Alice was adamant that she would leave the scales behind when she joined the school. However, she agreed to being weighed weekly at the school and would continue to have appointments with Gina every two weeks. Her final statement on the matter was, 'I know I have to maintain my weight.'

CHAPTER 7

Letting Go

As Alice prepared to leave home for boarding school I realised that she had been treading water for the last nine months and that we were now going to find out if she could swim. Although I knew it was essential to keep moving forward, it was terrifying jeopardising our routines that had kept Alice well. Inevitably we had spent so much time together over the past three years that I knew I would miss her tremendously. However, she showed no signs of regretting her decision and again I could only admire the determination she displayed towards the next phase of her life.

For the next two years the responsibility for Alice's illness transferred from the professionals, Alice and me to, finally, Alice alone, but the process was neither smooth nor easy. Although she was blissfully happy at her new school, her weight continued to fluctuate. When at her worst she was threatened with another admission by the consultant at the unit; at her best she made enormous strides forward towards leading a more independent life.

The entire process was nerve-wracking. When her weight dropped significantly Alice rejected any considera-tion of readmission, but in order to avoid this she had to endure spells without sporting activities, or periods when she came home each day for a month or two rather than board. I found the attitude of friends and family frustrating; it was difficult to get them to understand that it was the nature of the illness rather than Alice being 'very naughty again'. But deep down I had colossal feelings of guilt and irresponsibility that I had ever encouraged Alice to embark on a course when it seemed to be proving to be detrimental to everything she had achieved. Nevertheless, she rose to the challenge each time in order to regain her hard-won independence.

It was an extremely fine balancing act between letting Alice go and letting go of Alice. Too often she would say, 'I'm responsible for myself now, Mum, I know what I'm doing,' when it was apparent that in fact she was not managing well. Without the professionals' input it would have been all too easy for Alice to fool herself – and probably me – that she could lead a full life without continuing to tackle her anorexia. My part yet again was to implement their rules and to reassure Alice that in the long term it would be worth it.

Apart from discussing my anxieties about her health, Alice was disclosing fewer details of her life and I needed to respect that she was indeed growing up. How best to support her during this time proved a dilemma for me. In a typical week she would spend four nights at school and three nights at home. At school she crammed in every aspect of the school curriculum that she could – work, sport and socialising – and bluffed her way through her eating idio-syncrasies with some extraordinary stories including lactose intolerance, allergies, and so on. However, it was difficult to know whether at home it was best to treat her still as an anorexic or to continue to urge her on along her route to normality. In some ways I think it was a relief for her to come home and have a break from initiating the discipline required to maintain her exhausting new life away from home, however much she enjoyed it.

Alice's goal continued to be to attend medical school, and she knew that to succeed she would need excellent A levels, but, equally as important, she knew she would also have to be in control of her illness. Hard work had never been a problem for her but she needed constant reminding that brainpower required as much food as a netball match. It was a demanding combination and was not helped when periods of stability were disrupted by the transition of school terms to holidays and vice versa.

Towards the end of the first year Gina commented, 'Alice is flying by the seat of her pants', which absolutely summed up the anorexic part of Alice. Although her intentions were good, her tendency was to reduce the agreed amount of daily calories, and so she was still experiencing tremendous problems with her body image and maintaining her weight. She was a gutsy little soul, but the anorexic mentality often beat the logic of requiring a slight weight gain to ensure healthy ovaries and bones. Her headmaster's report, however, was glowing: 'she is already making a positive impression as a trainee prefect. I agree that she is a natural leader of others, and I am looking forward immensely to all she is going to do in terms ahead … she is a delightful young lady. If I could choose anyone to look after me if I were ill, it would be Alice! Her cheerfulness alone would make me feel better! . . . nobody deserves success more than she does.'

Alice had also recovered so much of her lost teenage years. She had acquired a boyfriend, expanded her social life and eaten food in unfamiliar homes, and her periods had returned, if sporadically; in fact she was really in most ways a typical 16-year-old.

Now I had to decide which way I was going to go with her. Should I resign her to a limited anorexic life, or encourage her forward? I had always received unasked-for opinions from others and now was no exception. One was that medicine was a ridiculous career for Alice to pursue and I should prevent her from even contemplating it, but my view was different. I knew she needed something to aim for – she simply was not going to eat enough unless there was a purpose. During her holidays she worked in the local hospice and she had received an impressive report from her seniors: Alice cared, she was diligent and responsible.

At the end of her academic year the consultant who had been treating Alice throughout her illness would either discharge her or refer her to the adult unit. I respected him immensely; over the years he had patiently negotiated his way through Alice's maze of objections to particular plans of treatment and had always been prepared to change tactics. As Alice had progressed, so the atmosphere at meetings had become less tense, and we had laughed when he suggested that if plan 583 didn't work we would then move on to plan 584. Now the clock was beginning to tick against us, but, under his guidance, Alice began to reduce her medication slowly, and the responsibility of weighing Alice and adjusting her food accordingly was passed on to Alice and me. No doubt Alice's ambition to go to medical school gave her an enormous incentive to succeed.

Having to make her university application was the first time that Alice met head on the implications of having suffered from a 'mental illness'. Her personal statement had to be good, and I found it heartbreaking when in fact she was advised not to put down what in fact she regarded as her greatest personal achievement: overcoming anorexia. It did little to help her overcome the shame, embarrassment and stigma that went with mental illness. Ian understood this well: he didn't share with anyone except me the problems he was experiencing with his panic attacks.

Alice's next hurdle was the medical history questionnaire. She was extremely apprehensive that her disclosure of anorexia would prevent her application from going any further and decided to ask her consultant if he would be willing to write an explanatory letter to the admissions tutors. It gave a totally honest account of the three years during which Alice had been under his care and ended: 'We do know that anorexia nervosa is a chronic illness and that it is likely to be some time before it can be said that Alice is completely free of it. However, as with other chronic illnesses, the path to success is learning to control the illness and lead a normal life. I would say that Alice has shown determination and strength of character for quite some time now and shows every sign of being able to achieve this ... I would be very hopeful that she would be able to manage a medical school course and life as an undergraduate from October 2005.'

Alice successfully completed her two years at school, building new friendships along the way. She had always been encouraged by both the medical and academic staff, who eased our path enormously by allowing us to adjust our schedule as necessary.

Olivia and Kier announced their engagement and we spent the summer preparing for the wedding. Alice, however, spent a month backpacking around Croatia; it was the biggest risk yet. She came home in time for the wedding – brown, smiling, a little thin, chuffed to bits and with a place waiting for her at medical school. I gradually accepted that although I could keep Alice stable, she needed an environment away from the memories and routines of home to enable her to take new steps forward.

The last date in my diary at the end of that hectic summer was our final appointment with the consultant. It was a surprisingly short and straightforward affair. Sadly, Alice was underweight again, and I wished that all his efforts could have been evident on the day of her discharge. However, his team of experts had given Alice and me every possible opportunity to manage whatever lay ahead. He gave Alice a hug and wished her every success for her future. As I closed the door he said quietly, 'This is quite big isn't it?' I replied that it was closing the door on the biggest chapter of my life.

Alice very quietly and effectively took control of her eating habits, and slowly but surely she regained the weight she had lost during the summer. And that is where we are today. Recently I asked Alice, 'Do you ever think you will be able to eat what we eat?'. Her reply was, 'Did you ever think I would be able to eat a meal on my own?' Sometimes it is all too easily forgotten just how much she has conquered in these past five years.

CHAPTER 8

Crossing Bridges

My thoughts on how I would conclude have varied enormously during the time I have been writing this book. Sometimes we have taken more steps back than forward, and at other times more steps forward than back; in between there have been long spells of wondering which way we were going to go. I know I am extremely fortunate in having a child who was prepared to tackle her OCD and risk leaving her anorexia behind, and now Alice is 18 it is apparent that she has taken many more steps forward. Had it gone the other way, I doubt I would have completed our story.

Before Alice's illness I had read those typical magazine articles recounting tales of anorexics and their extraordinary weight loss, and I quickly reached the conclusion that either the parents must be very stupid or their children very spoilt, but then, lo and behold, I get my own very special anorexic child. As an optimist I chose to believe that something good comes out of something bad. The bad is obvious, but on a good note I have been lucky enough to meet some exceptional children, parents and professionals who in turn have provided inspiration, understanding and expertise.

I am now able to answer many of my own questions. 'Was I doing everything wrong?' Not everything but quite a lot. 'Is anybody else finding this as excruciatingly difficult to manage as me?' Yes, once I had the opportunity to meet parents and share their experiences. 'Why wasn't Alice improving as some of her fellow patients?' In time I realised that she was actually improving more than some of her fellow patients.

To some extent we think she will always have an eating disorder – 'normality' has been a tricky one. In order for Alice to find it, friends and family have had to forgo what they could reasonably have considered normal. And finally 'support' – finding my way around this word has been the focal point of my days for the past five years.

My mistakes are obvious but at the time they were impossible to see. I let Alice do everything that the books warned I mustn't: she took control of her eating, she took control of my kitchen, but at that stage I hadn't read any books. But then I continued to blunder on, I was slow to find the correct professional help, and I was influenced by the stigma of mental illness. I allowed Alice to manoeuvre me when I hesitated in telling the professionals the full extent of the horrors at home. During the early days of Alice's admission I allowed her 'treats' when she came home rather than sticking to the tight regime set by the unit. And so the list goes on, but at the time I thought I was 'supporting' Alice.

I was slow in realising the complexity of support. It has needed adapting throughout Alice's illness to provide whatever was needed at the time. Support has embraced firmness, consistency, encouragement and, most of all, trust, reassurance and love. Love has been a constant throughout, but the

game has been learning when to juggle the other compo-
nents to Alice's benefit.

What else have I learnt the hard way? That there are no short
cuts; Alice at her worst could be extremely devious; if I was
angry this only left Alice feeling more inadequate and guilty,
but, conversely, praise needed to be approached carefully; she
also needed a very structured day, as her worst scenario was
sitting at home waiting for the next meal; exercise required
constant monitoring; any changes in the routine needed to be
discussed and agreed beforehand; as Alice began to improve,
meeting other people with the same condition bothered her –
anorexia is a fearfully competitive illness. On a positive note,
anticipating problems on her behalf, encouraging her to meet
her friends, find a job and have something to aim for have all
boosted her motivation. From the appointments with the
cognitive therapist Alice learnt that to survive she was going to
have to take some controlled risks – some have worked and
some have not, but that is the essence of risk.

It is extraordinarily difficult to relate to guide books and
put into practice their advice when it is your own child,
whom you have known all your life, that you are dealing
with. They suggest that conversations with your anorexic
child should be approached calmly and with understanding:

> You have told me you have some concerns about your
> health. You have noticed that you are not sleeping as
> well as you once did. Your hair has become thin. Every
> time you wash it, handfuls seem to come out. I wonder
> whether this might have anything to do with your
> weight loss. What do you think about that? (Janet
> Treasure, *Anorexia Nervosa: A Survival Guide for Families,
> Friends and Sufferers*).

It is asking an enormous amount of a parent firstly to accept that their child is so desperately ill and then to master this new form of communication. The theory is right, but putting it into practice is agonisingly difficult.

Alice and I have developed our own 'in-house' lingo. It has taken a long time and I still make mistakes. I am sure Alice would say that my most irritating word is 'just' – 'Might you just have an extra orange juice?' – but we can now discuss any problems that occur and how they might be sorted out. Alice has taken full responsibility for her condition but she does occasionally ask for my support if something is worrying her. I have yet to find an answer to her concerns with body image, which is the final major hurdle for her to overcome. I have intentionally avoided giving any explicit details of Alice's weight throughout the book. It is an immensely private issue for Alice; no doubt some anorexics will have weighed less than Alice but in some macabre way I feel that parents share the same competitive element as their anorexic children. All I can say is that Alice was breathtakingly thin.

'Why did it happen?' is Alice's least favourite topic and a question that I have asked myself over and over again. There are many possible explanations, but after endless soul-searching I have decided not to blame myself for her illness. She was and always will be hugely loved. I am sure she would agree that she had a happy childhood that, though not perfect, did not warrant the hell that she has put herself through. Alice once offered that 'it rained at the wrong time and weeds grew'. My feeling is that although Beth and Jenny were old enough and independent enough to cope as our lives changed, Alice, perhaps with the assistance of a rogue gene, was unable to.

We are still as close a family as we were before the onset of Alice's illness. Beth and Jenny have been wonderful and extremely accommodating in accepting a back seat during the past three years. Alice is in the fortunate position that her older sisters have largely been independent throughout the duration of her illness. Had she been the oldest, with younger brothers or sisters with their own demands, it would have been impossible to give her the amount of time and attention she has received. On the other hand, perhaps it would have forced her to adapt more than she was asked to do.

After working for a year in London Jenny decided that she would take a year out and make one last bold attempt to apply for veterinary school. While she cooked and cleaned on the ski slopes of Austria she received a letter from Cambridge accepting her application – joy of joys! Beth continues to move up the marketing ladder and was even sent to Miami to collect a 'Global Award' which she found highly amusing. Although we are scattered, we keep in close contact. Alice has seen her father on a couple of occasions since her discharge but she has yet to spend a weekend with him.

Bridges have been crossed too; the animosity between Ian's family and mine has been largely resolved, and genuine friendships have formed between the children.

And, finally, Ian – he deserves a medal. He has encouraged me to finish this book, allowed me to disclose some very personal information on the understanding that throughout I have been honest to everyone. He has endured the most turbulent four years both with work commitments and our problems. It has been a testing combination; farming has been as depressing to Ian as Alice's illness has been depressing to me. I am sure that during heated moments, many a good man in the same situation might have said that he had quite enough problems of his own and left me to sort out my own mess. Ian has been wonderfully loyal throughout but undoubtedly he would say that the stresses and strains have left the pair of us feeling old, fragile and exhausted.

I know I have changed. I am no longer the easy-going, go-with-the-flow person that I was, and I have given up trying to keep everyone happy all the time. Perhaps the biggest change is that I am organised and punctual. However, Beth, Jenny and Ian often ask where my humour has gone. Actually, I think it is returning, but in all honesty life hasn't been very funny for a long time.

Financially Alice's ill-health has been a burden. I am hugely fortunate that throughout the past four years my pay packets have remained constant, though my hours in no way reflected this. My mother financed a car to replace my old banger that broke down on too many occasions delivering Alice to the unit during our early days. Getting Alice on the road to recovery has increased my mileage from an average of something under 10,000 a year to closer to 20,000. My kitchen has not survived the incessant kicking it received during the jumping era: the drawers are either missing or hanging off their hinges. Ironically, an anorexic has been expensive to feed. We have certainly indulged in 'retail therapy', and Alice has never suffered the lectures her sisters received pointing out the financial demands of their social life. In fact my motherly words of advice have been more on the lines of, 'Go out, have a great time, drink too much and don't work too hard!' Beth and Jenny know that on a financial level Alice has received far more than either of them, but apart from the occasional cryptic remark have accepted it with good grace.

Writing this story has largely been a healing process for me: before I could begin to forget the nightmare of the past few years I needed to remember them. It has become increasingly apparent as our tale unfolds how fortunate I have been in so many ways. My family, Ian and his family, and our friends, have been exceptional in their love, patience and support during this journey. Our trump card was having the great good fortune of living within the boundaries of a most remarkable NHS adolescent eating disorders unit. Without its continued support after Alice's discharge from inpatient to outpatient I am sure we would have found ourselves once again on its doorstep, out of our depth.

The pivotal point has been Alice and her momentous decision, of which she wrote in her letter to 'Anorexia my Friend': 'I need to decide which I want more – you and your thinness or life and its decisions. Although no-one believes me, I choose life.' My job has been to encourage Alice in every conceivable way that she has made the right choice. My mistakes during the perilous journey are obvious; perhaps my successes are learning from my mistakes and continuing to do so. Kate Chisholm, while recounting her own anorexic experience, in *Hungry Hell*, suggested the importance of 'having a reason to eat' rather than 'having to eat'. I believe this is hugely relevant. It has taken a long time to get there but we now have pleasure putting the emphasis on the days ahead rather than the meals that need to be incorporated into them.

Alice is insistent that she is in control of her illness. In many ways her cards have fallen well recently and I have yet to see how she will cope with real disappointment. The more she expands her life, the more susceptible she is to the rigours of 'normality', but she welcomes the challenge. My thought at the start and end of every day is 'Where are we with Alice?', but it is not there every hour of every day as it has been. Alice has now been able to achieve a degree of freedom from anorexia, and I can only hope to celebrate this freedom as it develops.

PART TWO

Alice's Story

Introduction

When I first learnt that Mum was writing our 'story' I felt hugely anxious that she would become completely over-taken by the memories of the past five years. It seems a strange worry to have, and putting it into words feels even stranger. A massive wave of guilt overwhelms me when I think back over all that has happened, as I know that although the diagnosis is attached to my name it has been Mum who has been with me every step of the way; a commitment that I know has come at a great price to her own life. I worry that the scars of the past will always play on her mind and that she will always question 'Why did this happen?', probably to a larger extent than I ever will.

In our search for control we have both come to learn an enormous amount about this illness, other cases and their strategies. Although we have put a huge amount of effort into leaving the past behind us, Mum and I frequently fall into conversations about the illness – remembering times of disaster, progression, relapse and triumph. I often wonder whether both our minds will always be occupied with this illness, and whether we will always need the safety mecha-nism of remembering how far we've come in order to keep going.

It took me a long time to bring myself round to reading Mum's account of it all, though I think it was other people's fears that going over it all again might do me harm that deterred me more than my own. For me, reading the book would mean seeing it through another pair of eyes and therefore confronting the pressures and difficulties that I have forced on someone else. I have always found it difficult accepting that it was ultimately I who did place such enormous pressure on those around me and therefore I have a tendency to use the phrase 'the illness'. On that note it will quickly become obvious that I have a big problem using the term 'anorexia'; even with my close encounter I have rarely ever used it, referring to it as 'The A word', or simply 'it'. I have no doubt that a psychoanalyst would have a field day with that alone, but nevertheless it's just not a favourite word in my vocabulary.

Another of my pet hates is the use of analogies and metaphors – a good example being Mum's ideas about 'Planet Anorexia'. As you can probably imagine that was a phrase I just loathed! Over the years I have met a number of different therapists who all seemed to share a fondness for analogies, so I suppose it was from this context that I have learnt to associate them with madness. If I was sitting in a meeting and someone would say, 'It's rather like ... shooting ducks at a fairground', my mind would wander adrift then, thinking that this is totally stereotypical of 'therapy'. It made me question what my teenage friends would think should they overhear what was being said – surely they would think I was completely potty?

From what I have said so far, it has probably become obvious that I have had, and most likely will always have, a problem accepting that I do suffer from an illness. I have no idea why this is; I sometimes wonder whether it is because of my fear that people will think I'm boasting or parading my problems in an attempt to attract attention. After living in a unit surrounded by ten other people with the same problem, competition quickly arises; I have learnt that talking about low weights and diet is often more dangerous than it is beneficial. For example, in the unit patients often used to talk about the lowest weight they ever reached and it was almost as though the person who had reached the hardest bottom of the pit was the winner and deserved the most respect. When I first arrived there these conversations fascinated me and I won't pretend that I wasn't trying to be a contender in this lethal competition, but now I have progressed to the other side, weight and diet are both exceptionally private issues to me and, as a result, I don't talk about my 'scales history' with anyone, except of course with Mum in our attempt to stabilise where I am now.

Where am I now? After years of trial and error I'm just about in control of my eating disorder. I live a life in which my days are more about working towards where I want to be in life than working towards getting a life. It sounds like a wishy-washy answer, I know, but I use the phrase 'just about' because although my body's healthy I can't pretend that to an outsider my eating habits would look totally 'normal'. I still rely on the scales from time to time to show me what the correct portion size for meals should be, I continue to avoid eating most dairy products and other fatty foods and I prepare my own meals away from what my family eats. As I said to someone who knows my history, my eating habits would suggest that I am not cured of an eating disorder yet; however, from very early on I was always told that control is the cure for this illness.

When it comes to looking in the mirror, I don't know if I'll ever be satisfied with what I see. Even at my thinnest I could never see what the problem was; to me I still needed to lose more weight. However, I have learnt to live with the constant feeling of being overweight, and, for me today, knowing that my body is healthy and that my family and I can lead normal lives means more than being deathly thin. So control is what I have. Sometimes Mum asks whether I miss certain aspects of normality or if I crave foods that I once enjoyed but now avoid like the plague. The truth is that I'm happy at the moment, even with my restrictive behaviour, and I don't really see how eating roast potatoes will make my life any more complete.

After finishing reading Mum's part of the book I found that I wanted to write something to try to describe what it was that Alice, I, was thinking during those times when I seemed totally devoid of feeling. Like Mum, my intention in finally putting pen to paper is hopefully to help other people in a similar situation to ours to understand more about both sides of this illness. I also hope that in writing this I will be able to express the gratitude that I feel to my family, friends and the professionals, whose tireless efforts have been invaluable in getting my life back on track. At times I may seem to have taken their help for granted but I hope that the following proves, despite how it may have seemed at the time, that I was and always am aware of how much they have all done and continue to do.

CHAPTER 1

Tapping my Toothbrush

Home for me has always been an exceptionally happy place, mostly because of the relationships that I share with Mum and my two older sisters, Beth and Jenny. I don't remember if it was before or after Dad left that we became so close, but there isn't a moment in my memory that strays far from four having fun together. Despite being the youngest of three sisters I have never felt at all left behind or excluded, and although I couldn't always do what they were doing at the time, being the youngest definitely had its perks. Of course, there was the odd healthy teenage row and tantrum, and boyfriends came and went, but overall I have always felt safe and secure in my family.

I have instinctively scanned Mum's and my writing for an early sign of the rocky road to come, and I know she does the same, looking for any mistake that she might have made or for that time when she can pinpoint 'That's where it all began.' But I have never understood what it was that might have triggered the problems I've had. I prefer to believe that it may have been of genetic course rather than environmental, perhaps because this way it avoids anyone having to question whether they did something wrong. As for a beginning to it all, the obvious marker was when I as 11 years old and a long-term boyfriend of Beth's noticed me doing a funny routine with my toothbrush on the basin before I went to bed. He had a friend with an obsession problem and that's why he picked up on it. Before he jokingly asked me about my bedtime routine I had never really even thought about what I was doing. Without even being aware of it, I had completed the routine every night for as far back as I could remember. When Mum first asked why I tapped my toothbrush on the basin in that particular way I could only answer, 'It's just the way I do it.' And I suppose that's where it all began – tapping my toothbrush on the basin.

I have never been able to explain logically the reasoning behind my 'rigmaroles', as they have become known in our family, but put very simply they are a series of routines that I had to complete in exactly the same way every time, or else my anxiety would shoot to the roof with the fear that something awful would happen to my family. Another, more seemingly logical example of one of my obsessive routines was checking the iron before I went to bed at night. The reasoning being that if I missed the routine just once, that might be the night the house burnt down with Mum, Beth or Jenny inside. Therefore, to avoid the long-term agony, I must not be lazy and miss the routine. But soon the number of my routines rocketed and the justifications for doing them became more and more illogical.

During the phases of my obsessive-compulsive disorder (OCD) – as it was later diagnosed – I wasn't thinking about why I did my routines, they simply became habits. It was only when I didn't do them that I encountered the fears behind them and, of course, as soon as I didn't do one and the fears came I would simply complete the routine in order to relieve my anxiety. You can probably see the lethal cycle arising. Before too long the routines started to revolve around my lucky number, which was four: just to be extra safe I should do each routine four times to ensure nothing bad would happen. Once a routine popped up there was no eradicating it – it would have to be done that exact way every time. My rigmaroles infiltrated my daily life in my every move; even walking into rooms had to be done four times in exactly the right way (the right foot leading, hitting my hand against the door frame, reversing out and then coming in again). Of course this was very noticeable to those around me; it must have looked as though I was caught on camcorder and being rewound and played over and over again! My rigmaroles swamped me with anxiety and frustration.

The first time that Mum suggested I talk to the GP about my rigmaroles I felt so embarrassed about having to go to the doctor for something 'mental' that I refused. But everything came to a head one morning when Mum left me to get dressed and after 20 minutes I had achieved nothing more than putting on my underwear and was stuck repeatedly opening and closing the cupboard doors when she walked into the room. I can still feel the overwhelming frustration – unable to move on, no matter how many times I said to myself, 'Come on Alice, just leave it alone.' I think the frustration arose because I knew inside that realistically nothing bad would happen just because I didn't press the doors shut four times. I had lost all control. I felt totally defeated, and this time, when Mum again suggested that we see the GP, I was relieved at the thought of finding a solution, so I agreed.

I can't say that after our appointment with the doctor my rigmaroles disappeared, but it did help enormously. The reassurance of a medical diagnosis – 'obsessive-compulsive disorder' – made me feel less 'abnormal', knowing that there were thousands out there experiencing similar taunting thoughts. I did take control of the majority of the routines; forcing myself to stay in others' company was my main strategy, using the embarrassment I felt about my routines to keep them under control and also feeling safer not being on my own.

Over time I've built up a mental barrier and I can now remember surprisingly little about those desperate times. The thought of pushing through that barrier rings alarm bells – I'm still too frightened of being overtaken by the same routines to take that risk. Even today I find myself becoming more anxious when I'm tired, and I still have a few sensitive areas where the pressure of routines plagues my mind. For me, contamination has always been a major bogeyman. My hands will always bear the burden of this: endless washing has dried out my skin, leaving them red and sore. My eyes have also endured endless rinsing, and I still worry that if I touch a bottle of bathroom cleaner and carelessly rub my eyes, I might go blind. I find it really difficult admitting that I still feel these occasional compulsive urges; after all, today I live a pretty independent and 'normal' life. However, it makes me nervous in case someone will challenge these final fleeting routines. They require consistent monitoring on my behalf and I know that even with my experience I probably will never be able to knock them totally on the head.

Once we'd got the rigmaroles under control, I remember enjoying being at school with my friends, and liking the routine of the school week. I had a very close circle of friends – Nuala, of course, being my best friend. Things at home had grown fairly quiet; Beth had left to go to university and Jenny was spending more and more time studying for her exams. The house was quite tense and I wasn't always sure where was the best place to be during the evenings, as Jenny needed peace and quiet for revising and Ian liked this time with Mum. So I often resorted to the sitting room, watching television with my back against the radiator. I would shut the door and stay there until it was time to go up to bed. However, Nuala frequently came over and I was at her house just as often, so much so that our families often joked that they each had another daughter.

It was during these months that Mum started to ask me whether I was OK because she had noticed me becoming more quiet and withdrawn. I didn't feel that anything was wrong and thought she was making a fuss out of nothing, and as a result I often got cross when she tried to encourage me to join Ian and her in the kitchen. On reflection I can see that my anger was probably a means of not having to confront a problem. The day at the London Eye stands as firmly in my memory as it does in Mum's. It was probably the first time that we had an argument about my behaviour. I remember scanning the huge range of sandwiches on the menu very closely when we went to a pub-style restaurant for lunch. At this time I had no idea even what a calorie was, but I understood that different foods had different amounts of fat. Until now I had always looked at food using my tastebuds as decision makers but now there seemed to be something else to consider as well. I decided to have a tuna sandwich, as I thought it was a 'healthy option' even though it maybe wasn't what I would normally have chosen.

I'm not saying that that day was the start of it all, but it is the definite point that I remember starting to think about food differently. I recall looking at the dessert menu and shutting off my brain to what my body was saying, making myself have a coffee instead.

Another of my early 'food' memories is from one of my annual trips to Cornwall with Nuala. We had been going down to stay with friends of Nuala's Mum every year since we were tiny, and now that we were getting older things were becoming more fun as we were mixing with other people of our own age more: going down to the beach at night, day excursions to other coves and having fun sailing Topper dinghies and trying to capsize each other. I remember that one afternoon after a day's sailing we arrived back on the beach and out came the tea and biscuits. Everyone else launched in but I declined, telling Nuala how impressed I was with myself because all I had eaten that day was a bowl of cornflakes at breakfast.

At the time my attitude towards food wasn't about weight. Before Mum took me to see my GP, after months of no periods, I had no idea of my weight; even when he weighed me I didn't take too much notice of the numbers he wrote down. Despite my ignorance regarding food – I didn't even know that the nutritional information for foods was printed on the back of packages – it was during the next year that things started to slip away from me.

Over the next few months I started to think more and more carefully about what I was eating. I remember asking Mum to spread the hummus in my sandwich more thinly and leaving out any biscuits or crisps that she might have packed for me. To those around me there was nothing to raise the alarm bells over; it wasn't as though I wasn't eating anything – more that I was being 'healthy'. To me, the months when it all went wrong fade into a blur and I have no idea of a timescale during which it happened; the only guidelines I have are the school years. To my mind this was going on during year ten – I was 14 going on 15. The next big thing to go was the Flora from my sandwiches; I couldn't see the reasoning for having both a spread and a filling and so asked Mum to remove that as well. I was still eating a normal supper portion in the evening at this point, so I can't blame Mum for not picking up on the problem any sooner than she did.

One school night I was staying at Nuala's house. The following morning Greg, her dad, packed me off with the same sandwich he'd always made for me. When lunchtime came we sat at our normal table in the dining hall all gathered around opening up our different clingfilm parcels. To this day I remember seeing my sandwich and feeling horribly nervous about the amount of butter spread between the two pieces of bread. I can't pretend that there was even a huge amount to spur my anxiety. I couldn't bring myself to eat the sandwich as it was, so I began scraping out the butter. I could see that Nuala was slightly offended by this, but even the confused faces of my friends couldn't make me stop and eat it normally.

My eating habits got more and more messy. I began to scrape out even the small amount of hummus Mum was now spreading. I started choosing 'diet' yogurts and these, too, were being left unfinished. From time to time my friends would ask what was wrong with my sandwich and I simply said, 'I hate the way Mum spreads it so thickly.' If they asked why I didn't have something else I would say, 'This is my favourite'; I had an answer for everything.

I don't remember ever having the intention of losing a lot of weight, and I didn't ever think I was overweight, but there were certain parts of my body that I was never overly comfortable with, particularly my upper arms, cheeks and thighs, as these had areas of flesh that I could grip. I don't remember having any cravings for the foods I was avoiding, or feeling hungry, no matter how much I reduced what I was eating. If anything, I started to feel more and more satisfied the less I ate. I became more energetic – pushing myself harder in gym classes and after-school activities. I was eating a normal supper portion at home, but I was taking longer and longer to finish my meal. I preferred to be on my own in the sitting room when I ate so that I was free to take as long as I liked.

Then came the changes to my suppers. Although I continued to eat a sensible portion, I was choosing baked potatoes and pasta and leaving behind anything that contained butter, olive oil or cream. I don't know how the transition came about but soon I was cooking for myself and eating the same thing most nights: baked potato with beans, or pasta with tomato sauce, tuna and sweetcorn. I think I opted for these 'safe' meals as they circumvented any arguments with Mum about how much butter or oil she was using to cook supper.

Soon I discovered the nutritional information on the back of food packages. I only scanned the labels for the difference in fat and was starting to build up a mental database of the variations between foods. I remember stalking up and down the aisles in Tesco picking up every brand of product. I wasn't even aware of how long I was taking or if anyone was watching me. For some reason I developed a keen fascination for recipe books and cookery programmes.

I wasn't hungry but felt a sense of satisfaction knowing that I had knocked out all the high-fat ingredients that everyone else was still eating.

Having no bathroom scales at home at this time, I have no idea how much weight I had lost or even how much my appearance had changed. I can remember during one gym class my teacher had returned after maternity leave and she remarked about how much thinner my legs looked and that I ought to be careful. However, her warnings didn't make me think about what was happening; if anything, I felt another wave of achievement, which spurred me on further.

My periods had stopped a few months before this time but no one, not even me, had linked their absence with my eating habits. Even when I was taken to the doctor and he asked how much weight I had lost I replied, 'Very little', and to his question as to whether I was losing it intentionally I said 'No'.

Things continued to go further downhill; lunch at school was becoming increasingly stressful, as I started throwing away more and more food, which of course my friends were beginning to hound me about. At this time there was another girl in my year who was definitely struggling with an eating disorder. One day on the bus home I overheard two of her close friends talking about how thin she had become. One of the two said it was 'anorexia'. This was the first time I had ever heard of anybody having the illness, apart from in magazine articles. I didn't once think that what I was going through might be similar, but I started to watch this girl very closely. I felt strangely jealous when people commented on how skinny she'd become, yet when I looked at how painfully thin she was I didn't feel at all envious of her.

Meals were now becoming a battle at home; breakfast had mostly diminished and Mum was trying to persuade me to eat more at supper. I continued to dismiss the whole subject and wished that everyone would just leave me alone.

When Jenny worked through the list of different criteria for 'having an eating disorder' I tried to argue against every point, even down to saying that the fluffy coating I had acquired on my arms and face had always been there, when she pointed out that 'the growth of downy hair' was a symptom. I was confused and frightened. I knew that from now on things were going to get a lot harder.

We went back to see the GP who had been so reassuring with my rigmaroles. This time Mum didn't let me totally dismiss the conversation about my weight as I had done those few months before. She made sure I was realistic when I described what I was eating and how long my periods had been absent, and also made a stab at how much weight I had lost – she guessed it was around two stone. The doctor weighed me for the first time in years and suggested that I should start coming in every week to monitor my weight. More than anything he talked about trying to stop 'the downfall' before it got any worse, and about all that was in jeopardy if things continued as they were: school, sports, friends, health and fun. The doctor confirmed that I did have an eating disorder and I think Mum was relieved that her suspicions were correct. When I heard him, a doctor, use the term 'anorexia' I couldn't believe how out of hand the situation had become. I thought they were all making an enormous fuss out of nothing.

Over the next few weeks things got continually worse. I was throwing away more food at school (where Mum couldn't see) and arguments at home over food were becoming increasingly frequent. Mum invested in several books about anorexia, but I couldn't stand to see them about the house, as I felt that my case wasn't as severe as those she was reading about and that everyone was confronting me about problems that weren't really there. I had no idea that she was looking for more help, and when she told me that things couldn't go on as they were and that she had arranged an appointment with a specialist I felt terrified. Part of me was sure that they would laugh at the suggestion that I was suffering from anorexia, and part of me was frightened that I would be forced to gain a large amount of weight to stop everyone worrying about me.

During my period of speaking to the counsellor that Mum had arranged for me to see privately, we talked a lot about Dad and the relationship between Ian and Mum, and very rarely did food come into it. I found it easier to talk about our home without Mum in the room, as I feared that I was betraying her. On one occasion the counsellor took out a pot of different-sized buttons and asked me to select one to represent Ian, one to be me, and one to be Mum. This to me was the lowest point yet; I was convinced that I was crazy and couldn't believe that at 14 this was my life. Sometimes I felt that we were looking for problems that weren't really there, or just digging up the kinds of skeletons that were in everyone's cupboard. The meetings didn't counteract any weight loss and I was still getting into more and more trouble, but on the positive side they probably did help me to learn to open up more about what I was feeling.

CHAPTER 2

The Struggle to Take Control

I'll never forget the day that we first met the consultant psychiatrist and his team of experts. I was encouraged and reassured by the fact that the appointment letter had been addressed to Mum and me, as though I was going to be fully involved. Nothing had prepared me for what was about to happen. I assumed that it would be just like meeting a new GP, but as soon as we arrived at the clinic I immediately felt very uncomfortable about all the children's drawings on the walls – the stick men walking hand in hand under rainbows reminded me of the stigma that surrounds having a mental illness. I didn't want to be there at all.

Things got worse after the consultant met us in the waiting room. I was shown the room with its one-way window where the meeting would be held, and was also shown into the room behind the one-way window where there were four adults and endless wires and screens. I was too overwhelmed to take in the names of the strangers as they were introduced, but I met them all again many times after: it was the family therapist, the dietician, the clinical nurse specialist and the staff nurse. My talk with the consultant was to take place in the room with the one-way window, with his team of specialists watching and listening on the other side.

The consultant quizzed me about every aspect of my life: my home, family, friends, diet, self-image and more. He was too experienced for me to fob him off with my lies; he saw through me every time I brushed off a question with 'It's not really too much of a problem.' I felt as though I was totally exposed and couldn't believe that there was a team of people analysing my every sentence and move. I tried to look calm, to try to make them think that I wasn't panicking. I remember trying to smile and not look at the window, but the consultant touched on so many nerves that until now I had defended so carefully that soon I broke down in tears. He didn't immediately give me any feedback on what I said; for example, he didn't say, 'I think you're eating too little', but would say, 'Right, OK', and move on, but I knew the feedback was going on behind the glass. By the end of the first part of the meeting I felt completely exhausted. I had no idea what they thought about the answers I had given or how serious they thought my case was.

After the consultant's interview with Mum and me he left us while he discussed the situation with his colleagues. When he returned his opening sentence was, 'It is clear that Alice is suffering from anorexia nervosa and obsessive-compulsive disorder.' I couldn't believe that they could all have got it so wrong. In my mind there was no way my case was that serious; I wasn't thin enough and I ate too much to be anorexic. Clearly they all thought differently. Even after all that has happened I still question whether I really was anorexic, and whether I am today.

Straight after the meeting, I met the dietician who asked me to write down all that I ate in a day. Seeing it written down in black and white made me feel terribly guilty, as to me it looked like more could easily be cut out and that I was still being too greedy. I didn't admit to throwing away any food at school. We agreed on a few minor changes to increase my calories. I still wasn't familiar with calories but I didn't think the changes to be made would be too hard.

I decided that I didn't want to tell anyone at school about what had happened. I don't think I even told Nuala at that point; I was too embarrassed and thought they might laugh and say I was exaggerating. Without thinking about it I still kept throwing food away, and the changes the dietician had suggested went out of the window. My science teacher, whom I got on really well with, was the first to confront me about what was going on. One day after the lesson had finished he asked me to stay behind for a few minutes. He said that several other staff had mentioned how worried they were about me and asked whether we were dealing with anorexia. I tried to reassure him that I was on a straight-and-narrow path, but he didn't look convinced as I left the lab anxious because I had missed my precious gym class.

The French family holiday was disastrous for us all. I remember finding the water absolutely freezing and wrapping myself up in as many towels as I could find. I found it difficult to complete my morning exercise routine with everyone in such close quarters and I couldn't relax knowing I hadn't done it. I was arguing more and more with Jenny and Mum about food and could see that Mum was getting more uptight with worry. Jenny tried to talk to me about how irrelevant one glass of orange juice was and to make me see that I was heading for real trouble if I didn't start following the meal guidelines the dietician had laid down. I always promised that I would start complying, but every day I threw more and more of my cereal over the wall and the arguments got fiercer. My birthday supper was the worst yet – with the enormous gâteau that I couldn't eat any of. I felt awful about the restaurant's wasted efforts, and I realised that things were going to be much harder than I had expected.

Saying goodbye after the first week, I could tell that Mum was panicking. She looked exhausted and I felt terrible knowing that it was because of me. When I stayed with Miranda, I remember being terribly cold, bundled up in fleeces (it was June). She tried her best to keep track of my meal plan but I was beginning to tell lies and continued to exercise in private. Things weren't any better with Beth; if anything, they were worse, as she confronted me on how stupid I was being and told me that I was only cheating myself. I began to get frustrated with her 'interfering' and blazing rows would ensue, leaving us both in tears. Small routines of jumping had developed as a form of exercise and were getting more and more out of control. I remember Beth begging me to stop – but I couldn't.

When Mum returned she couldn't believe how quickly the situation had deteriorated. Rows accompanied every meal and her 'tight monitoring' of my exercise made me more irritable. I remember so little about the two weeks of work experience that followed, except for endlessly bending down to pick up pencil crayons off the floor as a form of exercise. At the end of the work experience, when Mum told me I wouldn't be going back to school, I was furious that she had gone behind my back. I couldn't believe that I wasn't allowed to go to school; I pleaded and cried but there was no shifting her decision.

At this time I was having two-weekly, one-to-one appointments at the clinic with a staff nurse, called Sarah, for MET (motivational enhancement therapy). In those sessions we talked about my self-perception. I felt enormously overweight. We discussed my attitude to foods and also how I was getting along with my family and friends. I realised that I completely misunderstood how much a person needed to eat to stay alive and healthy and had a fear of eating high-fat foods such as butter. I was surprised that people around me ate so much but didn't seem to put on weight. I found my talks with Sarah really helpful; she understood exactly what I was feeling and if I was ever struggling to find the right word to convey my thoughts she knew exactly what I was looking for. From her experience in dealing with people having similar thoughts, I felt less alone.

When I phoned Nuala to tell her what was going on, I asked her not to tell anyone at school other than our other close friend. She didn't sound shocked about what had happened and reassured me that she'd try her best to keep me up to date with the work I was missing. This was my biggest fear about not being allowed to go to school. I was terrified that I would never be able to catch up on all the lessons I had missed and might be put back a year at school. The summer holidays were coming up fast and I was determined that I would have to miss only three weeks of school and then spend the best part of the summer holidays conquering my problems.

Our other friend called me after the first day I was absent from school. It was a surreal conversation; we'd always been very competitive with each other and over the past months she'd started eating less, which made me worry that I was pulling her down, too. I couldn't explain to her why I wasn't allowed to go to school; I think I was too ashamed to admit that it was because I couldn't be trusted to eat enough food and that a school day was too strenuous for me.

My first morning as a day-patient in the unit is a blurred memory – as is much of the time I spent there. I remember carefully picking out my clothes – I chose the biggest things I had in my wardrobe so that the other patients wouldn't be able to see how much bigger I was than all of them. We rang the buzzer and one of the care assistants opened the door to us. He told us the code and it dawned on me that I would soon know it by heart. He said that I could take my shoes off and leave them by the door. I was surprised to see the row of shoes all neatly lined up – something I had never noticed before. It was a Tuesday and I was told in advance that I would be weighed when I got to the unit; I had been refusing to be weighed at home and so was once again clueless about my weight.

The other patients (all girls at this time) were standing in the waiting room in their dressing gowns and slippers and I couldn't believe how many there were. The unit had beds for ten full-time patients. The care assistant introduced me to the girls; some said hello, some smiled and others looked too consumed by nerves even to notice I was there. One girl was very chatty; she explained that she had been at the unit for only one day and that although it might seem scary now it really wasn't that bad. I noticed a hospital wristband on her minuscule arm and felt embarrassed that I didn't have one, too. At that point one of the girls came running out from around the corner in tears and zipped off back down the corridor towards the bedrooms, with the healthcare assistant behind her. The girls looked at each other. I felt sick with nerves.

Mum sat with me until it was my time to go into the clinical room. We watched as each of the girls was called in and then reappeared again a few minutes afterwards. Some came out looking totally placid and not wanting to give anything away, one came out smiling and the other girls hugged her to say 'well done' (I later learnt that she was leaving at the end of the week so long as she stabilised her weight), some were in tears and some stomped out in anger.

I was the last patient to be weighed that day; I walked terrified into the clinical room, where I met two nurses. I was surprised to see my name already at the head of a page in a book on the desk. I didn't know what to do so I waited to be told. They said that I would have to be weighed in my underwear and explained that some patients in the past had hidden weights in their clothes. I started to peel off my layers. I could no longer wear bras because the underwiring had started to cut my skin, but I was so relieved that I was wearing a vest and reasonable knickers! The scales were unlike anything I've ever seen. They had a base with a long stick, which had a box on the end that flashed bright red numbers. As I stepped on, the numbers changed from 00.0 – they climbed slowly and eventually stopped. The nurses checked the figure and wrote it down. I had never heard of being weighed in kilograms before and so had absolutely no idea whether this was a reasonable or low weight.

I came out of the room in a daze and told Mum what I weighed. I've always told her the changes from week to week ever since that day, so that she can have some idea of how I'm doing. The morning had been traumatic enough already and all I wanted to do was get back in the car with Mum and drive home, go back to my school and see my friends. However, I was called through to join the breakfast table and Mum got up to leave. I didn't want to be left and began to feel terribly nervous once again.

I had made my breakfast request the previous day after my final meeting with Sarah. I was put on a 700-calorie meal plan and was asked what type of cereal I would like, brown or white toast, what juice and what flavour jam. When I came to the table I saw that my place had been put beside the healthcare assistant (one sat at each end of the table). There were clingfilmed jugs and bowls all over the table. I did my 'sitting down skips' as discreetly as I could and sat down. My name was on several of the clingfilmed items. I watched the girls around me peel off the film and start pouring out their individual volumes of juices and reluctantly pull their carefully weighed bowls of cereal towards them, and I did the same. The girl next to me said that she thought she had too much cereal but the carer then reassured her that he had weighed it himself so she sighed and picked up her spoon.

Everyone around me had different additions to make to their bowls; there were labelled cereal bars, plates of diced fruit, flapjack, raisins and more. I noticed that the girls were mashing up their cereals into a paste and carefully spooning it around the sides of the bowls to avoid eating it all. I thought this was a clever idea and, though I had never smeared my food around my plate at home, I wasn't going to be the one here who didn't do it. I asked if I could change my spoon for a teaspoon but was told that I should try to break that habit in an attempt to get back to 'normal' eating.

I finally got through my cereal, after being asked to scrape up every last bit. Next came the toast. I remember feeling horrified at seeing a teaspoon of Flora and one of jam on a saucer with my name on it. I tried to explain to the carer that I couldn't eat any more. He looked at me sympathetically and told me that he knew it was hard but that I had to finish it before leaving the table. Shaking, I picked up my knife and began sliding my Flora around the plate. He shook his head and asked me to start spreading it on the toast. Breakfast that morning had taken me over an hour.

I left the table bewildered and went to join the other girls, who had finished before me, on the sofas. Justine, the other new girl, showed me how to fill in the supervision book. I had to write down the time I finished eating and what time it would be an hour later. Supervision took place after every meal, and for those who followed the rules and were moving forward it would slowly be cut down. During this time I wasn't supposed to use the loo but should I become desperate I would be escorted by one of the carers and asked to repeat the alphabet while the door was closed, to ensure I wasn't being sick.

At nine o'clock the other staff began to filter in through the sitting room and into the office for handover. I felt relieved to see Sarah walk in, but nervous to see the consultant follow shortly after. Next we were called into the morning meeting. One of the girls was still at the table finishing her breakfast with a care assistant. During the meeting Sarah took out the diary and read aloud what waited in store for each of us that day. I had three meetings: one with the consultant (as did all the patients on a Tuesday after being weighed), one with Sarah and another of the specialist nurses to talk about my diet and level of exercise, and finally a meeting with the cognitive therapist, whom I had never met before. School would be going on as normal.

Next the nurse asked who would be going with whom for 'walks'. I felt relieved at the mention of exercise but this was short-lived, as Sarah told me that to begin with I wouldn't be involved. She could obviously see the disappointment on my face as she quickly reassured me that it wouldn't be long before I was allowed on 'staff walks'. I soon learnt that there were two variations of 'walks' depending on how far the patient had progressed in the programme: those who could be trusted not to run or go off for miles were allowed 'peer walks' with other patients, but those who were not as far advanced would be accompanied by a member of staff ('staff walks'). Both types were carefully timed at 20 minutes and both took place twice a day.

My meeting with the consultant was very brief; he asked how I was settling in and how I felt about being part of the unit. I couldn't give a terribly enthusiastic answer with my stomach still stretched from my dramatically increased breakfast. However, I wanted to keep positive, as I was determined that my stay in the unit would be shorter than the estimate I had been given of four to six months. I was desperate to be back at school for the first day of the autumn term. The consultant asked me how I felt about my weight and told me that I had lost a lot more since my assessment. I responded that I still felt enormous and didn't feel I needed to be there. He took out a body mass index chart and began explaining how dangerous my situation was, but it didn't make a difference. I thought he had it wrong.

My meeting with Sarah and the specialist nurse was probably more daunting than with the consultant because they wanted to give me a large calorie increase. I tried to argue that I couldn't possibly manage what was already prescribed let alone more, but there was no shifting their decision. I was expected to gain 1.5kg a week and so my calories would be going up to ensure this happened. I wasn't allowed to participate in any exercise. I argued that until now I had been much more active at home. Surely doing so much less but eating so much more would make my weight balloon? They both tried to reassure me that I needed to eat more simply to stop losing weight, let alone to increase it gradually. My life was falling down around me. I wanted to get out of there. Inside I knew that there was no way I could do what was needed and I felt totally trapped and wrought with anxiety.

I was relieved to get into the classroom and try to give my brain a break from thoughts about food and weight. I launched hammer and tongs into the task of keeping up with my schoolwork. During my time in the unit I was forever being asked, or told, to sit down. I used to get extremely frustrated, thinking the staff were doing it just to spite me; I felt as though they had completely forgotten how a 'normal' person lives – occasionally they do stand up! So schoolwork soon became a sanctuary, it was something I could do sitting down without making me feel even more fat and lazy. During supervision time I used to write endless letters to my family and friends because I wanted to be doing something productive all the time that I had to be sitting down; the television had become my worst enemy, because I associated it with being a lazy couch potato, and I didn't want to watch a second of it. We arranged for my schoolteachers to send work in to me at the unit and some of them visited me regularly. Mary, the teacher in the unit, was fantastically enthusiastic and strongly encouraged my efforts to keep up with my own school's pace.

Different patients saw schoolwork differently: some were completely uninterested and didn't seem to care about what was going on beyond the unit, a few became obsessed with art and poetry and some, like me, used the work as a distraction. This resulted in a strange atmosphere in the classrooms. A few of us would sit quietly beavering away at the back of the room but there was always some form of covert communication. This became worse as the schoolwork set for us to do started to slow down before the holidays. With less pressure to keep up I was often distracted by conversations about food or gossip, such as so and so choosing to have a muffin for lunch – didn't they know that was nearly a hundred calories more than a Müller rice? Mary occasionally became irritated when we used her classrooms to discuss the things we weren't supposed to. Fittingly, it was in the classrooms that I learnt the most about different foods. It quickly became obvious who knew the most about food, and I soon began to home in on them, bombarding them with questions like which was the lowest-calorie supper option, or which had more calories, an apple or a pear?

Life in an eating disorders unit is the strangest situation I have ever encountered. How can you describe the atmosphere as ten anorexics sit down to an evening meal, or the conversations we used to have during our walks (I was able to take part in 'staff walks' after about two weeks as a day-patient). Professionals have asked me whether I found it beneficial or detrimental being in such a claustrophobic environment, surrounded by other people going through similar problems to those I was experiencing. My answer has always been that it was a double-edged sword: whereas it was a huge relief to talk about my thoughts and fears with people who understood, I think I 'caught' a lot of bad habits from life in the unit, such as the smearing, a consuming obsession with calories as well as fat, water loading to defy the scales, and many others.

I settled quickly into the routine at the unit. Mum would drop me off before eight o'clock in the morning, then it was the ever-growing breakfast, with supervision, meetings, school, walks, lunch, supervision, school again, more meetings, waiting for time to go by, the five o'clock meeting, stretch and tone, supper, supervision and then, finally, home. My days went incredibly slowly. I couldn't distinguish a Monday from a Friday. The only differences were weekends: with less staff working, we had no meetings and time passed by even slower. Thanks to my already established obsessive personality I was engrossed in rigid structure; every day had to be the same as the last. Every morning I dreaded that it would rain and stop me from going for my walk. If there were not enough staff to do stretch and tone, I would do it before I went to sleep instead. I was terrified that by missing out a single activity just once I would gain huge amounts of weight. It's hard to distinguish which of my obsessions were driven by my eating disorder and which by my OCD. My consultant has often questioned this and we both reached the conclusion that the two became lethally intertwined.

My rigmaroles must have driven the other patients mad. By now they had largely become focused on exercise. Every time I sat down I had to do a few skips on the spot, despite the staff telling me not to. It was also a known fact that I was exercising in the loos (larger jumps there). Having to sit down must have been hard enough for the other patients without having to do it while watching me hop about like a kangaroo.

With my calorie intake being continuously increased, I was jumping more and more. The staff at the unit were aware of my behaviour and were unimpressed. Soon I was no longer trusted even to leave the sitting room on my own. I was put on 'escort', and a care assistant would accompany me whenever I went into another room or to the loo. My jumping had completely taken over. I remember a typical Tuesday night sitting on the sofa in the sitting room trying to write a letter but being overcome with worry about what would happen in the morning when I stepped onto the scales. I had developed a close friendship with another of the patients in the unit. She was exceptionally quiet and I felt very privileged whenever she spoke to me. We talked about how much we wished that we could start this week again but this time comply with our own individual programmes – she wouldn't hide her food and I wouldn't jump. In our hearts we both new what the morning would bring: no weight increase on the scales – meaning another calorie increase and another wasted week. We were both caught in our own vicious cycles.

Things were becoming more intense as I was being more and more restrained, and there were few times when I could complete my jumping routines. I was still a day-patient, but my lack of weight gain had appalled the consultant and I was continuously being threatened with inpatient admission. Throughout these weeks I did everything I could to keep positive; telling everyone that I wanted to get out of the unit and that I had managed to knock out a few of my routines. I became incredibly frustrated that no one would ever congratulate me on my own small triumphs. I felt that they all expected too much of me and should be more satisfied with what I had conquered already. On reflection I can now see how irrelevant my 'triumphs' were. I was painting a positive image of a very negative situation. I can now see what they saw back then: nothing was really changing and I was becoming more desperate to hide this from them. My consultant and the family therapist were two who could not be fobbed off so easily. They knew what my game was and weren't having any of it – I grew to hate their meetings. They both spoke straight-down-the-line honesty and I feared that they would take Mum on their side, too.

Things at home were dire by this time. It was now just Mum and me in the house during the evenings after I got home from the unit. If she was at all late collecting me, I became exceptionally anxious and irritated that my routines would be disrupted. Ian had stopped coming for supper and Mum's life revolved around trying to stop me jumping. It took me three hours to have a bath and get into bed every night and the mornings were equally disastrous. Mum would look down at my red swollen feet and beg me to stop my jumping, saying that they looked crippled with pain.

She was right – I have never experienced pain like it. Hours of jumping and banging my feet as hard as I could for maximum stress on my body were taking their toll. I lied to Mum, telling her that I had seen the unit doctor and she had said that there was no actual damage beneath the skin, and promised that I would go and check in again with her the next day. Not once did I mention the pain I was experiencing to the doctor; I was terrified that if I did she would strap me down. The mental torture of not being able to do my routines would have wrecked what was left of my brain. Once, when I was walking with Sarah to a meeting room, she asked me if I was limping and I quickly answered that I hadn't noticed anything.

I can't explain how unreal my jumping was. The most excruciating part for me was not the pain, the exhaustion or the embarrassment but the frustration that I couldn't stop. Mum would always come and keep me company and try to persuade me to stop jumping, but nothing she said had any effect and blazing rows would often commence and both of us would have tears pouring down our cheeks. I didn't have the strength of mind to be able to cut down or end my routines – I would have had to face my fears about consequently gaining enormous amounts of weight. The staff at the unit were having a similar problem: they would knock and knock on the door of the loo but I wouldn't reappear until I had finished my routine.

Every three weeks a review meeting was held with the consultant to discuss my situation. It was normally me, Mum and Jenny, but Beth tried to make it whenever she could. Before the meetings I would try to persuade Mum not to be too negative; I bombarded her with my 'triumphs' in an attempt to cloud her desperation and hopefully prevent her from asking the consultant for any more help. I knew I was only hanging on at home by the skin of my teeth and begged Mum not to let them 'take me away' and make me an inpatient. I thought my main fear about becoming an inpatient was that I would no longer be able to do my routines. I now realise that my intentions all along were to avoid gaining any weight.

A common theme at these meetings was medication. The consultant strongly recommended that I begin a course of antidepressants to help me with my eating disorder and OCD. I always refused, despite everyone's encouragement, and I was adamant that I didn't want 'a drug' to take control for me – I wanted to do this myself. The consultant would reason that surely if I had a broken leg I would accept the aid of crutches, but it didn't change my decision and I would not be forced.

After three months in the unit my jumping had reached a climax. I had held Mum exhausted and terrified for too long and in my heart of hearts I knew I couldn't go on either. I was breaking every rule in the book: going on extra walks when I got home, exercising non-stop and being sick. I had devastated our home and Mum's social life, and affected her health as well. I knew that by the time the next review meeting came round I would have my final chance to remain at home. Mum wasn't going to be manipulated any more if things didn't change.

It was to this review that Dad was invited as well. I hadn't seen him for over a year and was exceptionally nervous about what would happen with all the family in a room together, let alone thinking about what the consultant was going to say. My relationship with Dad is more like the relationship I would share with a family friend rather than a father, even down to the 'we must meet up more regularly', though of course this never happens, for which we are both to blame. Despite spending so little time with him, I have always defended his name throughout arguments and have often been hurt to hear negative comments made about him.

I could hear Mum, Beth and Jenny discussing the meeting at home, reassuring each other that it was going to be OK. Beth and Jenny decided to help Mum write down all the things she wanted to say so that she could clearly describe what she was thinking and not be crushed by her nerves during the meeting. I was petrified because I knew they wouldn't let Mum write down anything other than the exact truth. This time I wasn't going to be allowed to put any emotional pressure on her to make the situation seem less serious than it was. I was furious with all of them, thinking that they were ganging up on me. I told them that they all just wanted to 'get rid of me'.

The meeting was everything I feared, and more. The extent of my jumping at home had been fully exposed, new restrictive rules were made and there was an enormous amount of tension between Mum and Dad. After Mum had worked her way down the list the consultant asked Dad if he was aware of this situation, to which he truthfully answered, 'No.' Dad's only involvement in my 'treatment' up to this point was the phone calls Mum made to keep him informed of how much worse I had become. Even after I left school and became a day-patient Dad hadn't called me, let alone visited. I was shocked to hear him go on to give his judgement: he said that Mum and the staff weren't doing what was right for me, and that we all had our heads in the clouds. What hurt me the most was Dad's final comment: 'Alice clearly doesn't want to get better.' He didn't know how wildly frustrated I became not being able to stop jumping; he didn't know how exhausted I was, fighting the same battles every day to eat what was demanded of me; and he didn't know how much I missed my school and my friends – he hadn't seen any of it.

The consultant informed us that he didn't have any beds available at that time but that one was coming up shortly and I would be admitted full-time if I didn't dramatically change my behaviour in the evenings. He gave Mum, Beth and Jenny the task of making me a strict timetable to divide the time between getting home and getting into bed. For example, at nine o'clock it was time to get into the bath, at ten past it was time to brush my teeth. I said that I hated the idea because I felt totally useless and pathetic, but inside it was more because I was aware of the mental aggravation that would swamp me when I didn't complete my routines. At the end of the meeting I ran out into the corridor to the loos, where I jumped and cried. I felt totally betrayed by Mum because she had been honest and I didn't want to talk to her.

I wasn't able to confront Dad about how much he had hurt me during the meeting, so when it was time for him to leave we said a restrained goodbye and he promised to phone more often. Mum, Beth and Jenny tried to talk to me for a while after the meeting but I was too angry and upset, and I had nothing to say to any of them then. But after they left I felt terribly alone. I knew I was being completely unreasonable and that their intentions were to help but I couldn't shake off the feeling of betrayal. The only words I spoke to them that night were to tell them how much more difficult they had made things for me, and that all they had done was to make me suffer more mental torture.

The timetable that they devised meant nothing to me. I felt more consumed by my rigmaroles and more alone than ever before. When Mum told the consultant that this new plan wasn't working we embarked on another strategy, this time working much more closely with the cognitive thera-pist to try to relieve my anxiety and help me to reduce the intensity of my routines step by step. I felt confident that with his understanding of OCD we would be able to make some ground.

The cognitive therapist had worked with many people who struggled with OCD. He could make me laugh even during the worst of times and I always felt that he was on 'my side'. Before this we had spent most of our meetings talking about my reasoning behind my rigmaroles. He had shown me a graph of anxiety against time and explained how I used my routines to relieve my anxiety more quickly than having to wait for it to fall naturally. One time, after I had explained my fears of contamination and said that even holding money made me feel nervous, he took a coin from his pocket and rubbed it on his eye. Another time he licked the bottom of his shoe! I was completely gobsmacked, but reassured. The next day he gave me a few coins to hold and then came and sat with me during lunch. I wanted to wash my hands but he persuaded me to hang on – sure enough, after about ten minutes my anxiety had gone and I no longer felt that I needed to wash my hands.

The cognitive therapist asked Mum and me to write down exactly what my rigmaroles consisted of. The plan was for us to cut down the number of jumps slowly and for me to rate my anxiety on a scale of one to ten immediately afterwards, then again ten minutes later, and so on, and hopefully we would see the scores descending. The first major problem was trying to describe my routines on paper so that Mum could keep track, but I started to get frustrated that she didn't understand the different variations and decided that I would keep track myself. For the first couple of days things seemed to be going well; I started to feel better in myself again, and I no longer thought the world was against me. Looking back, I know that my more posi-tive mood was actually a result of having fewer people nagging me about my jumping. I started to lie about cutting down my routines, but the tell-tale signs for Mum were that I wasn't any faster at getting into bed at night or leaving in the morning.

At the next review Mum didn't hide the truth that things hadn't changed. That very afternoon I was admitted as an inpatient. Strangely, I didn't feel betrayed by her as I had done after the last meeting; I knew she had given this final plan 100 per cent and had encouraged me all the way – by now I knew it was me who was failing.

I found the one-to-one nursing care total torture. If being away from home and always being watched wasn't bad enough, I was also put on to bed-rest, which was far worse than anything I had anticipated. I had to be on my bed with my feet up all the time, except during a few hours of the day when I was allowed to attend school. I was watched by a care assistant during the day, who would tell me to sit down whenever I got up, and during the night a nurse would sit outside my slightly opened door and make sure that I was not exercising.

For the first time I gave into my exhaustion and I felt pains in my body that I had until now blanked out. I discovered that I was totally terrified by my illness. It hit me hard, as I finally realised that I did have a serious problem. Now I was left to face the underlying issues that I had avoided confronting. I had to face my eating disorder and my ultimate fear of gaining weight head-on.

Those four weeks were the worst of my life. Writing this has made me see that even today the memory of it is still red-raw. I will always remember sitting on that bed in the small room, with the door ajar and a care assistant sitting outside, thinking to myself that I wanted to die. For the first time in years I missed the person that I used to be and also realised how much I had been missing my family and my friends. Dad called more often, but sporadically, and as things changed so quickly he was never up to speed and had not experienced enough to understand what I was going through. As a result he would ask painful questions about how much was I eating now or dive straight in with asking how my weight was. The worst feeling for me then was eating and waiting to gain weight, so for someone else to associate me initially with both of these increased my anxiety and confirmed that I had turned into a lazy lump.

In the past I've sneakily read a few pages of Mum's books on anorexia, which she refers to as her 'bibles'. I usually home in on the sections about food and meal plans with the same fascination that I have with recipe books. I am always amazed to read the foods that they suggest giving to people suffering from the illness, such as *pains au chocolat*, sausages, high-calorie muesli, macaroni cheese, meats with creamy sauces and even chips; and they suggest replacing yogurts with chocolate bars, ice cream, pies and pastries. I can't believe that they would honestly expect a person with an eating disorder to manage them.

In the unit a rumour spread about one clinic where on Tuesday nights fish and chips were bought locally and all the patients had to finish a portion of this 'more normal' food. One patient who was in hospital with me at the time had actually stayed at this clinic and when we asked in horror if it was true she looked filled with shame as she confirmed it. At least our unit designed the menu plans and ingredients with our futures in mind; instead of forcing us to contend with our worst food fears (high fat content) they opted for foods that we would be more likely to continue eating by ourselves and incorporate into our diets after we left the stability of hospital.

Every week after being weighed and discussing what changes would be made to our calories the patients met the dietician. Before these meetings we would all sit looking at the 'conversion sheets' wondering how we were possibly going to incorporate the changes – for me always calorie increases. When you're eating nearly 4,000 calories a day already it's a huge challenge to find any gaps to sneak in that extra 200. Some patients decided to condense their calories, opting for the high-calorie but less bulky way. For me, I knew this wasn't worth the mental aggravation, so my meal plan looked and felt enormous.

I became more devious at the table, hiding raisins and other food in my mouth and spitting them into tissues, dropping food on the floor or sneaking it into my pockets. As a result, certain foods were taken off my meal plan and exchanged for more bulky items; so, for example, at breakfast I was no longer allowed raisins but had to eat two pieces of fruit on top of everything else.

Being admitted as an inpatient meant spending a lot more time with the other patients and unit staff. I found it hugely difficult to see patients I had said good luck and goodbye to only a few weeks before walk back in through the door looking terrified at the thought of having to do it all again. It stirred a mixture of feelings inside me, including the realisation that being discharged from hospital in no way meant being cured: if anything it marked the start of the biggest challenge yet to come – keeping our new lifestyles going without the staff telling you to. In contrast, the arrival of a new patient stirred up dangerous competitive urges among the patient group; for example, asking each other, 'How different do I look from the new girl?' Seeing the size of their meals in relation to mine made me realise how much I was eating now compared to when I had first arrived at the unit – what a long time ago that had been.

The group of patients who had come into the unit at around the same time as me all seemed to be progressing, leaving me the straggler left behind. The repercussions of my 'rule-breaking behaviour' were not only that my estimated stay at the unit was forever being extended but also that many of the patients began to avoid me. They witnessed me exercising in the loos and hiding food in my pockets and watched me go home every night knowing full well that I broke every rule there, too. I had alienated myself: the other patients had grown to see me as a danger because I abused the system that they had all learnt to respect. I felt desperately lonely as the other patients formed a very close circle. My closest friend (the quiet girl who hid her food) had been spending more time away from the unit by now because her eighteenth birthday was looming and she was keen to be discharged rather than referred on to an adult clinic.

In one of my later sessions with Sarah I tried to explain how excluded I felt from the patient group. There had always been strong friction between me and another patient in the group and as I started to surface from my spell on bed-rest I began to realise that she was at the heart of this exclusive patient group. She was always catching me out jumping and reporting on me making other mistakes. I couldn't stand her breathing down my neck and bringing everyone's attention to my battles.

All my feelings came to a head on the first day that I was finally granted peer walks; it had been arranged in the morning for me to go with the other girls after my meeting with the cognitive therapist. I found the sitting room empty and when I asked the nurse where everyone was she told me that this girl had asked for them to leave early that day. I knew she had done it on purpose to leave me behind. Sarah asked me if I thought I was being bullied by the other patients. I hadn't intended to get anyone into trouble and I didn't want to make any further waves within the group, so I said no and told Sarah that it was just petty feelings that I needed to get off my chest. Perhaps it was.

The one advantage to being in the unit was that I got to spend more time with Gill – one of the healthcare assistants at the unit. On my first day she had confronted me about having tissues under the table and, for some reason, from that point on we 'clicked'. She was probably one of the strictest members of staff: sitting next to Gill at the table meant scraping your plate dishwasher-clean! However, she did seem to talk to the Alice I used to be rather than the Alice I had become. We made each other laugh and she seemed to understand that I never intended to end up where I was. During my time on 'one-to-one' and on bed-rest we would sit together for hours talking idly about how she was decorating her house, our friends and family, and anything else that would keep my mind distracted and help to make those endless hours of torture pass more quickly.

CHAPTER 3

Finding 'Normality'

As the days turned into weeks I finally stopped jumping. The school term had started once again, it was my final GCSE year and I was hugely relieved to see the work and deadlines start arriving. I spent the afternoons in my room, still on bed-rest, reading textbooks, filing and refiling my work, and writing letters. Inevitably, doing so much less exercise did begin to take effect and finally my weight began to rise above the starting line. I grew more and more uncomfortable in myself, and my conversations with Sarah were entirely occupied with trying to combat my feelings of being overweight and my negative body perceptions. Sarah would print me out endless articles on the physiological dangers of starvation and being at a low body weight; she knew I worked best on a scientific, factual level. The threats of infertility and osteoporosis still plague my mind today.

Another feature of our sessions was to test how wrong my body perceptions were: she would first ask me to make a circle out of string that I thought was the same size as my thigh, upper arm or waist, and then by using the same piece of string she proved to me how much I overestimated the size of my body. I never derived a huge amount of reassurance from these exercises as I was always terrified that I would underestimate the sizes and Sarah would have to extend the length of the string to go round my thigh. I was sure that one day I would catch her out and she'd be shocked to see how big I had become. It never happened, but the fear was so real that I've never done the exercises since then.

However, for once I did start getting 'rewards' for the results of my efforts, and I was finally allowed to resume having walks. They were shorter than before but I felt a huge wave of achievement and relief that I was finally doing something 'right' and receiving something back in return.

As I came off bed-rest and returned to unit life – but this time complying with the rules – I started to rebuild my relationships with several other patients in the unit. Although we talked a lot about food and calories, I now found that I could talk to them about 'teenage' things, too. I started to get the giggles again and even became a little mischievous – we would have water fights in the bathrooms, take stupid photos and do impressions of the nursing staff.

Mum suggested that maybe Nuala could come in and visit one weekend, and although I was apprehensive about her seeing me eating I had been missing her company, so I agreed it would be a nice idea. I hadn't anticipated the shame I would feel as she entered my new world. She brought a couple of letters with her from friends at school, and looked surprised when I asked where people thought I had disappeared to. I was disappointed to learn that most people had simply guessed what had happened.

Just before leaving, Nuala asked me how long I thought it would be before I would be starting back at school. The reminder that that world was going on without me hit me hard and persuaded me to take my pace of recovery up a gear. I realised that the time I had spent in the unit going backwards had been 'real' time to everyone else. While I had been jumping my friends had been going on holiday, having relationships and generally having fun.

As time went by I started to think more about what I wanted to do should I ever get out of hospital. In my mind I had convinced myself that eventually one day I would wake up and be cured, but I now realised that I needed to work hard to make my life different. I could either live my life in and out of hospital or I could take the risks of recovery and actually do the things I had once planned.

For me, being what is considered a 'healthy' weight – and there is much dispute about what this is – means living a life of discomfort, not only in the physical sense (the awful feeling of always feeling full and overweight) but also being incredibly uncomfortable about how I look. I worry terribly about what people think when they see me. With friends, family and those who know me personally it's the fear that they will think I've possibly gained too much weight. With strangers walking past me in the street I wonder whether they see me as an ordinary-looking individual with a 'healthy' covering of insulating fat. The truth is that there are very few body shapes that I look at and can think that I would be happy with if that's how I looked, too. Normally, when I point out my ideal figures to Mum she'll look worried and tell me that they're too thin.

I was determined to show my consultant and the family therapist that I wanted to take more control, and was finally granted the chance to spend several hours away from the unit at home on a Saturday afternoon. Having 'supervision' with Mum at our kitchen table made me see that I had been living in a world consumed by an eating disorder and that in many ways I had lost track of how 'abnormal' my life had become. For the first time in months humour cracked into our lives, and Mum and I talked about how bizarre our lives must seem to total strangers: a chunk of malt loaf on the scales on the sideboard, our afternoon planned out for us by a family therapist and counting down the hour before we were allowed to leave the table.

However, it was accompanied by a sense of longing for the relaxed atmosphere and routine that we used to have in our home. Mum was stricter than I remembered, and there was no way I was going to find a way to 'bend' the new rules. She was exceptionally rigid on no smearing, no getting up and down to get this or that during supervision time, and walks were carefully timed to 20 minutes. To be honest, the rebellious streak in me was still tempted not to abide by *all* the rules, but on reflection I can admit that what Mum called giving me a 'helping hand' was a huge relief. Even though I wasn't jumping any more it was still a battle to stick to my path of going forward, and maybe I wasn't as ready to take full control as I wanted to believe.

The combination of both Mum's and my revised efforts turned out, against all odds and in contrast to what the professionals thought would happen, to be successful. Even though our time at home was anything but relaxed we had bridged the gap between life in the unit and life at home. Over the next few weeks I started to spend more and more time rebuilding my confidence and independence in our home. Although Mum still accompanied me when I went to the loo, we started to relax a little more about making plans for our afternoons, we spent less and less time with the family therapist and started making decisions for ourselves.

My first night at home was a tremendous occasion for us both; not only had we managed three meals on our own but we had established a new routine where 'going upstairs to bed' didn't mean commencing on the next phase of jumps. That night as I climbed into what Mum called my 'cotton-wool bed', for its powers of recuperation, I felt a huge wave of satisfaction. I had no idea how it had happened but somehow I had finally found some light at the end of a very long dark tunnel. During all my time in the unit I had never been able to look beyond my hospitalisation. Whether this was a protective mechanism to prevent me from becoming too depressed I don't know, but I could never ever imagine being able to leave. Yet now here I was at home in my bed. I was not cured but things were beginning to change.

My personality slowly started to return. My relationships with the other patients flourished as they saw another side to me than the devious, negative Alice of old times. I made great friends with two patients in particular, a girl and a boy. The three of us came from very different backgrounds: Sean from inner-city London with his various face piercings and cartoon sketches, Tasha with her love for shopping, clothes and going out, and me the country bumpkin with her books. For some reason we totally clicked. We started to work towards our goals together; we would all try our best to 'put in a good week' on the scales so that we would be allowed out together into town or home for longer at week-ends. We longed to get out of the 'madness' and rigidity and start getting back into normality.

One evening Tasha and I arranged to try our first meal out in a restaurant together with our Mums. We were looking forward to setting a stepping-stone in place that we might be able to use later on when socialising with friends.

The meal went well. I thought carefully about how it would look to those tables around me if I mutilated my food – picking apart every inch of chicken for rogue strains of fat – and I tried to avoid dissecting every forkful. Having another patient with me while I ate this alien, unweighed meal was a huge help. Doing it together made me feel less anxious about the unknown size of the portion, as realistically I knew it wasn't going to do anything dramatic to Tasha's weight, and with her there in front of me I applied the same logic to myself.

The next big event I remember was meeting up with a group of my close school friends for an afternoon in town. Nuala had made all the arrangements. I couldn't imagine how much I must have changed from what they remembered. They were all boys and I had the feeling that they understood very little about what had happened. Fortunately, no one said how much 'better' I looked, as I have a tendency to misinterpret 'better' as 'fatter'. We strolled around the shops and even went into McDonald's (though I didn't eat anything), and the afternoon was another step in the right direction.

I've never talked about anything to do with my illness with any of my friends except Nuala. I don't know why but I have always felt a sense of embarrassment or shame about what happened, and as I result I tend almost to try to pretend that it didn't really happen. It surprises me when I think about it; how could we be so close and yet they know so little about the hardest time in my life and the ongoing challenge I still experience every day. I suppose it's because I've shown them only the Alice I want them to see. It's an Alice with the same positive outlook, or what some might call a lack of reality, that I tried to summon up in front of the professionals to hide everything that was really happening inside. I managed to convince them all for a long time that I really did want to get better, buying me more time and independence to work towards my real goal, which was putting off the weight gain for as long as possible.

It's not like that today, I'm not lying or hiding anything from my friends, but when I'm with them I try to forget everything that went wrong and concentrate more on what I want them to think when we're together: do I want to be the Alice caught up in her own issues, talking about 'what happened to me in hospital' or the Alice who's in with the best of them and game for having fun?

Another breakthrough for me was when Ian's daughter Olivia and her boyfriend Kier came to the unit to see me and we sat outside in the sunshine and played a board game. We were all cheating in our normal family fashion, and at one stage I stopped and realised that for about 15 minutes I hadn't thought about food. However, 'snack time' sneaked up on us and I faced the dilemma of whether to wait until they left and eat my snack later, to avoid them seeing me eat, or keep to my usual time and routine but have it with Livvy and Kier. I decided that I would feel more uncomfortable if I ate it later, so I asked the nurse if I could have it at the table with my visitors.

Out came the Jaffa cakes, fruit and juice. I felt exception-ally embarrassed about eating the Jaffa cakes. One problem I had about eating was my loathing for the jelly layer in the middle of Jaffa cakes. I had found a way of pulling them apart so that this tiny circle of jelly was left until last, giving me the perfect opportunity to put it in my mouth so that it looked as though I had eaten it, but once I left the table I would spit it out into a tissue or just put in it my pocket if using a tissue would draw too much attention to what I was doing. It was a great trick, but it turns out that I wasn't as crafty as I had hoped; having to chat to Livvy and Kier at the same time made my task much more challenging. About a year ago they told me that they had seen the jelly moving around in my mouth as I mumbled my words. Mum caught on pretty quickly, too, and soon I was being asked to open up my mouth for inspection before leaving the table – the jelly trick had been squashed!

I finally got my head around the idea that if I was going to stay out of hospital I would have to accept that people were going to see me eat. After coming to terms with such horrors it seemed reasonable that I would be allowed to set a date for my first day back at school.

The Thursday night before my first day back at school I felt sick – not only because I felt stuffed full from supper but also because I had so many feelings racing round inside me. I couldn't wait to be back in the classroom with all my friends, but at the same time I knew how easy it would be for one stupid remark to throw me off-course and land me back at square one. I didn't sleep a wink. In the morning I felt as though my mind was a million miles away from my body, watching myself put on my new school trousers, pack my books into my bag and eat breakfast. I couldn't believe that this day had finally arrived. I felt as though I was starting everything again from scratch.

It was a surreal experience to feel so nervous about something that I had been waiting for for so long. Stranger still, for the first time since my admission I actually longed to be back in the security of the unit, rather than screaming to get out. For months all I had wanted was my old life back and yet now that I had come so close I missed the safe, consistent routine that I had established in hospital. I knew everyone there and they knew me, I didn't have to give any explanations or dodge around any awkward questions. Perhaps this explains why it was that so many ex-patients had to be readmitted to the unit only a few months later.

No matter how much I wanted to return to school and normality, it was going to be a huge challenge. I was going to take responsibility for eating everything I should and not over-exercising; I was going to have to rebuild the relationships that had lain dormant for nearly six months with my friends, teachers and so many others. Although a large part of me wanted to run away back to my usual routine and setting, another part of me was determined to make this work. I had experienced too many dire times in the unit to entertain thoughts of staying there long-term.

As Nuala and I approached our form room I felt as though I hadn't been gone a day – nothing had changed. Nuala opened the door and led the way in. Everyone was turned around in their chairs talking to the people who were sat at the desk behind, and our tutor was at the front rustling through some papers. We snuck in and sat at our old desk. I felt safe and almost cocooned in a secure nest. I had people I trusted all around me. It was just as I had hoped: so far we had slid in and no one had made a big deal of our entrance.

After this point those first few days and even weeks back at school all seem to fade into one in my mind. All I know is that all my anxiety about someone saying something about how much better I looked or wanting to know why I had been absent from school for so long amounted to nothing. Workwise, I was still on schedule to take the GCSE exams in the summer. I was relieved at how easily things slotted back into place after so long away.

The transitional period between being at the unit and being back at school full time was the hardest time to keep everything together and stay up to date with my school work. Being back in the classroom at school two days a week made it difficult to organise exactly how much work I would need to cover during those three days that I spent in the unit. It began to get quite confusing and very stressful to remember what work and books were where and which lessons I had missed and which I had been present for. I longed for some stability and was finding it increasingly difficult to explain to people why it was that I was in school for only two days a week. No doubt the explanation of 'going back to hospital' had started to crop up in more people's minds and they probably gathered that I still wasn't totally 'cured'.

The constant feeling of being unsettled made me keen to try to bring forward my discharge date to as soon as possible. I wanted this 'split personality' period to come to an end and be allowed to concentrate on getting back into my old life rather than keep going back to the hospital and having to attend meetings, which I began to feel were dragging up all the feelings I was trying to suppress. The idea of 'suppressing' these feelings (of diet and being uncomfortable about my weight) probably sounds very unhealthy and as though I was putting off dealing with the issues at the heart of my illness. But I was beginning to feel 'talked out'. I felt that I was just going round and round in circles. I didn't know why it was that I had developed these problems and to me the best strategy for the future was to get on with my life and deal with new challenges as they arose.

Mum, on the other hand, seemed to grow more and more nervous as I began to start talking about leaving the unit. Although I could understand her fears of how easily everything could go wrong again and of losing the safety net of the unit, I had little enthusiasm for the meetings that we were still attending. I tried hard to avoid seeing the family therapist, as I felt that the meetings were turning more into counselling sessions about our family situation with Mum, Ian, Beth and Jenny, and less about dealing with an eating disorder. I began to feel as though I was being put under a magnifying glass and people were digging too deeply to find the heart of my problems.

I can't deny that the thought of leaving the unit unnerved me; I would be leaving behind a tremendous proportion of my life, saying goodbye to great friends, shutting off that familiar and safe routine and embarking on life on the outside. I worried enormously about what it meant to leave hospital: did it mean that I was now a 'healthy' weight (which to me was still an uncomfortable thought in itself); did it mean that from now on I would be expected to eat completely normally – fish and chips and everything? A further worry was that should I ever have slip-ups, make mistakes or misjudgements that resulted in weight loss, would everyone think I was failing and send me straight back into the hands of the professionals? Nevertheless, I had managed to re-prioritise my life; being back at school with my friends, preparing for exams and looking further into the future were more important than any of the risks that accompanied leaving the unit.

My time at the unit tailed off rather quickly. After returning to school, changes started to happen much more swiftly at the unit. I was allowed to start preparing my own meals under supervision, my supervision time after meals was cut back, and I was trusted and left to my own devices. Foodwise, I was still 100 per cent reliant on the scales when putting meals on the plate and still using a specific meal plan to stabilise my weight within the 2kg target range decided by my consultant. I started now to take more responsibility for managing my meals, accepting that at around three o'clock I would need to eat a snack and whether it was me or the nurse who remembered it first it was going to happen anyway, so I might as well think about it myself. My meal plan was still very large; months of jumping had meant that my calories had had to spiral very rapidly at the beginning and that my body had adjusted to this large energy intake, so I would need to maintain it at that level to avoid losing the weight I had finally gained.

Once I started eating my lunch in the school instead of in the car with Mum, having Nuala with me was a tremendous help. I felt guilty tearing her away from the lunchtime buzz in the dining room and the company of all our friends, but she never once faltered or even suggested that she minded staying with me. I was hugely grateful to her for being there, and I knew that she wouldn't say anything confrontational or threatening like 'Why can't you just take a bite rather than picking it apart?' or 'Wow, that's a big lunch.' However, that didn't stop me having pangs of embarrassment that at 16 years old I needed to ask my best friend to sit with me alone because I didn't like eating with lots of people around me and I couldn't be trusted yet to eat on my own.

A few weeks after returning back to school I crawled over the bottom end of my target range and my discharge date was finally put in writing. I would need to gain a little more weight to get to the middle of my range, which, according to my consultant, had the advantage of giving me some leeway for the natural fluctuations that a normal person's weight experiences from week to week. To me, the concept was torturous: being in the middle of the target range meant weighing more than I 'had to'. Before I even embarked on the process of stabilising my weight I was nervous that my OCD would be reawakened with the fear that should something change (exercise levels or what I was eating) my weight would change dramatically. Sarah was on hand to rationalise all my fears and, even though I was worried that voicing these fears to her might mean that she would step up my level of supervision, I had learnt to trust her and her definition of support. It was arranged that after being discharged I would continue my sessions with Sarah and together we would work through any new challenges as they arose and she would advise me on how to stabilise my weight.

Although I felt relieved that I had finally reached my target range, I can't deny that at times I did feel slightly envious of the new patients as they arrived: they were beating me in that lethal competition to be the thinnest. I knew these thoughts were incredibly unhealthy so I tried hard to concentrate on how much more freedom I had won myself. Mum was fantastic in helping me to remember that at the end of the day I was coming out on top because I was finally getting my life back on track.

I remember leaving the unit very clearly — it was all so final. Even though I would still be returning every week to meet Sarah, I would no longer be part of the patient group. I knew that I would still see the staff when I went back for my appointments but it was as though they were handing over the responsibility to me and Mum, and that from now on, rather than being central players, they would be spectators watching how we did. I knew I would see Tasha and Sean again but I found it very upsetting knowing that if all went to plan we would never have our close circle again. Gill wasn't working on my discharge day, but as my 'key worker' and close friend she made the trip in just to watch me go. I find it incredible that even thinking about it today still makes me feel slightly sad: I had been so miserable there yet somewhere amid all the agony I had found security and reassurance.

The biggest task leading up to my departure was finding a suitable gesture that could possibly reflect the enormous gratitude that our whole family felt towards the staff. Mum came away with the clear intention of helping to raise funds to support summer activities and facilities available at the unit, while my idea was to make a collage of photos taken during the happier times I had spent there. I hoped that it would be something that might bring hope to future patients and that it would also commemorate my patient group so that we would never become forgotten names of the past.

The car ride home was a silent journey; whether it was nerves or sheer disbelief, neither Mum nor I could find any words that could possibly express what we were feeling. I never truly thought that it would ever happen; for so long I could see no further than a life obsessed by finding new ways to avoid the pressure of everyone around me forcing me to gain weight. Although the sensation of being 'well' enough to go home was incredibly agitating, I so wanted this next risk to pay off.

It's strange considering how vividly I remember leaving the unit on that last day, when the next phase, like so many others, is almost entirely lost from my memory. I often hugely overestimate how long it's been since I was admitted to the unit, or since I stopped taking my medication. It terrifies me that, in relative terms, it wasn't that long ago. The harsh reality that I was still jumping even after leaving the unit brings some drifting memories back to mind: jumping in Nuala's bathroom in her house before going out for an afternoon, Mum coming upstairs to chat to me while I bathed and got ready for bed – the list is in fact endless. It reminds me just how much further we had to go after I left hospital.

Being back at school full-time was exhausting. My friends moved through every day at a pace that at times I could only watch in dizzy wonder. By nine o'clock at night I was totally shattered and there was no way I would be able to go out or even catch a wink of night-time television. I found the demands of coursework deadlines and the rate at which our exams were approaching hugely stressful and consuming; all I wanted to do was keep working, do that one extra question, read that one last revision book. Mum's alarm bells started ringing, as she could see the challenging targets I was setting for myself.

Everyone kept trying to persuade me to lighten the workload a little: 'After all, you have been absent from school for over six months.' But the thought of people using my eating disorder to justify my attaining lower academic achievements only spurred me on to work harder. I have an incredibly competitive trait in my personality, and I wasn't going to let myself fall to the bottom of the class. The advantage of my determination to get the results I wanted was that schoolwork once again provided a haven away from the harassing thoughts about food and weight. Sitting down with a book in front of me was one of the few times I would be still and not agitated about what was going on inside me.

Exercise-wise, the freedom to take part in sport during the week rather than rigidly depending on two 20-minute walks a day helped me to move away from strict routine; nevertheless, I was adamant that I had to do at least one sporting activity every day.

Throughout the week my anxiety about my body image and how much I was having to eat would accumulate and I always looked forward to my sessions with Sarah, so that I could relieve some of the tormenting feelings that were building up inside. I began to grow more uptight about people telling me that I was looking 'well', as I was obsessed that they could all see me growing larger and larger. Every week I came in saying that I knew I had gained weight and I couldn't shake the inner feeling that my thighs had got wider or that my neck was looking chubby. The scales told a different story: my weight was in fact remaining relatively consistent with a few negative slip-ups here and there. The same issues went round and round: how was I going to become less reliant on the scales to weigh my food, when and how was I going to broaden my diet to a wider range of foods and, the most challenging, how could I address my distorted body image? It became clear during these sessions that I was suppressing a huge amount of tension; I was taking every comment deeply to heart and reading an inner weight-related meaning behind most things that people said to me. However, Sarah always worked through the sessions with limitless patience and logical counter-arguments, such as, 'How can you be overweight if your periods still haven't returned?', or, 'What do *you* mean if you say to someone "You're looking well" ?'

During holiday time, when my school routine was broken, my weight would drop. I always seemed to over-estimate how much more exercise I was doing at school compared with what I would be doing at home. As a result, I became more restless at home and also reduced my diet – not a good combination – so inevitably I would lose weight.

Even today the word 'holiday' doesn't fill me with excitement, as I know that it means a lot of empty days and inevitable tensions about filling those days with something to keep my mind busy.

While I was in the unit I often felt incredible anger and frustration welling up inside me about how restricted I was in every aspect of my life. I felt horribly guilty venting these feelings on Mum and the professionals, as they were only trying to help. I knew that trying to explain what it was that was making me angry would only make me even more frustrated. I began to write my negative feelings in a black book that I had been given as a present, firing out everything that I was feeling inside but that I didn't want to talk about. I've never allowed anyone to read it. After leaving the unit I started to write in my 'black book' less and less. I know that whenever Mum saw me writing in it she thought I was having an enormous battle and became nervous that perhaps I was slipping downwards. Sometimes I think I used this association between my book and tougher times to remind people that although I seemed to be coping on the outside, this was possible for me only by controlling a mass of feelings within.

One particular entry in the book stands out in my memory. It was the afternoon that Mum and Jenny finally said that I couldn't go on my school ski trip. I remember feeling totally heartbroken and gutted. Once I realised that

Mum wasn't going to budge on her decision I went straight upstairs and found my black book – I pushed my pen down so hard scrawling everything that I felt inside. When I reread the entry I was surprised to see that I had for once vented all my anger on my illness and myself – not once did I blame Mum or Jenny. I was furious at myself for continuing to lack independence.

During the holiday in France that Ian arranged for his daughter Heidi and us I realised how food-orientated I still was despite leaving hospital several weeks before. Evening meals out in a restaurant were particularly difficult for me. I would start to worry about supper from about three o'clock onwards and by the time we finally sat down I found that I was already beginning to struggle with the mental battle against cheating and finding some way to eat less than I was supposed to. It was at this point that I finally accepted that the ski trip would have been a disaster – without Mum there to reassure and guide me on what to order, I would have been entirely lost.

This constant learning process continues even today. Remembering how it was that I've come to be more independent around food and managing new challenges as they arise brings back a mesh of many disjointed memories, and I find myself having to rely on Mum's account to remember what happened where. Sometimes I find it incredibly frightening how much I have forgotten. Looking back at photos taken before things started to go wrong, I hardly recognise the girl I used to be: on the one hand I can't believe I lived with myself looking that big for so long; on the other hand, I can't believe how simple life once was.

The next big step I can locate in my mind was Sarah's suggestion that I should look for a weekend job to try to alleviate some of the anxiety as to what I could do to fill in my time away from the school routine. Waitressing appealed to me the most, as it wouldn't mean sitting on my bum all day worrying about not doing enough exercise. However, I was still completely phobic about touching nightmare foods like butter, cream and oil. Chopping the butter was torture − I hated the feeling of it on my hands and once I had finished it took a lot of washing until I was satisfied that it had all been washed away and I could relax about touching my face or unconsciously biting my nails.

During the summer holidays I picked up more shifts at the restaurant. However, I dreaded the end of each shift, as all the staff would sit down together and eat their lunch of leftover 'goodies' − roast beef, roast potatoes and chocolate cheesecake. It's not hard to guess why this wasn't my favourite time of the day! It was always difficult explaining to the staff why I didn't want even just a taste of anything, and I came up with endless excuses. This aside, I was really enjoying the busy nature of the work and the satisfaction of earning some money of my own.

Saying goodbye to Sarah when she went on maternity leave was very strange; neither of us could predict where I would be in terms of my recovery when she came back to the unit, and it raised a lot of questions inside me about how long I would continue to need help to manage my eating disorder. However, the change from Sarah to Gina gave me a new jumping-off point and accelerated the rate of things changing and improving. I found it easier to break old habits and finally found myself moving out of the rut. I moved away from wanting to talk about the same issues each week and I realised that I had been afraid to move on and talk about other things with Sarah in case she thought I was suddenly cured and no longer needed her help. With Gina there was a fresh slate and I felt less ashamed moving on to talk about new problems that were arising.

We talked a lot about my relationships with my friends and me managing a life doing everything they were able to do. She encouraged me to take risks and not to dismiss anything as impossible. I was still incredibly reluctant to follow her idea of finding new ways to measure out my food portions, however; for instance, using dessertspoons or measuring cups as an intermediate step then moving on to using handfuls. For a long while I backed away from taking the plunge – it was so much easier using the security and accuracy of the kitchen scales. My weight was still shifting around my target range.

One day I mentioned to Gina that Mum and I had been looking at the idea of me going to a boarding school for sixth form. The concept excited me enormously. Ever since I was small I had dreamed of boarding school. What appealed to me the most was the idea of always being surrounded by others, tennis courts awaiting just a hundred metres away and the fullness of a day – knowing that I would very rarely be left with nothing to do.

When I told my friends about going to boarding school they couldn't believe it. For the first time in a long while I was the one taking the biggest risk and going that extra step. Most of them were going to pass along the fairly natural route of going to one of the two sixth-form colleges in town. Although these colleges produced exceptionally good academic results, I knew from Beth's and Jenny's experiences that the colleges could become pressure cookers, putting an enormous amount of stress on producing high grades. Mum and I shared the same fears that if I went to such a large, competitive school I would become lost in a world of pushing myself to the limits on every level and have little chance of anyone around me even noticing that my health was slipping downhill once again. For me, the supposed benefit of moving on to the college with a familiar group from our school was actually a disadvantage. In my school no matter how independent I became I would always be 'the girl who had anorexia'. I didn't want this reputation following me around for the rest of my life and determining how I 'should' act around food. I dreaded that every day for the rest of my life I would always be associated with eating disorders. I wanted a clean slate.

Things ticked along at home; I continued to use scales to weigh my meals and was just as reluctant to try using them less, even though I knew that in just a few months' time I would be starting at the new school without them. At times I became incredibly frustrated at how difficult I found it to move on; I felt as though more and more of my life was leaking away from me and I still couldn't find the confidence to do anything about it. Even though Gina hadn't known me during my hardest times in the unit, she would still draw lines of continuation to show me just how far forward I had gone without even noticing. She pointed out how different my life was from the time when I needed someone to sleep outside my room to prevent me from exercising in the night, how I was back full-time at school eating lunch with my friends rather than in the car with Mum, how I had a job and faced my fears of touching butter and cream, and much more.

Achieving good GCSE grades was another hurdle that I had to jump, and I began to lose hope of achieving my target grades when I thought of the amount of time at school I had missed. However, my science teacher came to my rescue, encouraging me to keep aiming high because he thought I still had the potential to get the grades I wanted. My main fear going into the exams was whether or not I had built up my concentration spans to stay alert for up to three hours. I remember coming home absolutely exhausted after each big day, but I'm sure my friends all felt exactly the same.

The last weeks of school were a sad time for everyone. For me they were the last few weeks I would ever spend being at school with Nuala, and, although I was hugely excited about my new school and the fresh faces, I was going to miss her terribly.

The evening after our last exam was a big night in everyone's diary, it was the school prom. We'd watched older brothers and sisters get glammed up and now it was finally our turn. For some reason the prom was exceptionally important to me; it was the ideal chance for me to make an impression and show everyone around me that I was more to remember than 'Alice with the eating disorder'. The night itself was everything I had dreamed of. I had my friends, a corsage and a new beginning in front of me. I felt totally at peace with myself.

CHAPTER 4

Strawberries Minus the Cream

During the summer my weight had fallen just below my target range, but remained stable at this level. Knowing that I was a slightly lower weight helped me to feel more relaxed and less driven to be on the go all the time. Gina and Mum strongly urged me to gain that final bit of weight to be within my range, and, eventually, with my consultant, they increased the pressure to the point where I had to get up to the agreed level and learn to live with the discomfort I experience at being a 'healthy weight'.

When we made plans to repeat our annual summer holiday to the South of France, I asked Mum to pass the message on to our friends joining us that I really didn't want everybody mentioning how much better I was looking compared with last year, despite people's kind intentions. Even though Nuala was suffering from a tummy bug and intense homesickness during the first week, she was nevertheless reliable as ever and sat by me for all my meals. I was becoming incredibly uncomfortable about so much time around the pool; no one really wanted to go for walks in the baking heat and Mum watched me nervously when I started swimming lengths. My holiday nerves built up inside me. I followed my instincts and made reductions where I could – buying ice lollies to replace my Jaffa cakes and assuring Mum that they contained the same number of calories, pouring away milk and orange juice, and basically abusing any opportunities when I was trusted with more responsibility. As the week progressed I became more anxious about my weight, I felt enormous and I was convinced that my body was getting bigger. I started being sick after meals – not to the point where I totally emptied my stomach, just enough so that after eating I didn't have the horrible sensation of being so full. I told myself that this was to be only a 'holiday habit'.

Inevitably, that week when I stepped onto the scales Mum's face dropped. I told her about everything, as I didn't want to get caught up in the cycle where my calories increased dramatically and I then felt that I had to continue being sick to avoid consuming them, which only led to even larger calorie increases. From my experience in the unit I knew Mum could be a support in overcoming this – by my telling her the truth she would eliminate the opportunities I had to go and be sick, thus avoiding me needing to have further calorie increases.

The old routine was reinstated, with supervision back on the scene for an hour or so after meals, and whenever I went to the kitchen or the loo someone would come and chat to me. I wanted to put things right and prove to Mum that I wasn't going to be overtaken by the 'unhealthy' part of my brain, what we called the 'green mush', and so we agreed that I would be reweighed after four days. With our tighter regime I started to regain some of the lost weight. I had seen how quickly I could convince myself to revert back to old ways, but I had also learnt that Mum and I were now equipped with the know-how and trust in one another to correct my mistakes.

In the weeks that followed I wanted to show Mum that I could handle more responsibility. Slowly she began to let the reins loosen a little, and agreed to let me go down to Cornwall with Nuala and her Mum for a week. She made it very, very clear, however, that I would have to be weighed every three days, and should my weight fall below the bottom of my target range I would be on the next train home. Nuala knew the routine well by now and was there to help me 'be honest' when preparing my meals and sticking to everything on my meal plan. I think Nuala's family and our other friends down there were too nervous to remark about anything to do with my health for fear of upsetting me, and as a result no one said anything other than that it was good to have me back on the beach. I ended up having the most fantastic week; I felt more like the Alice of old without being surrounded by so many 'knowing eyes' waiting to see how I managed my next meal.

Back at home I told Mum and Ian that I wanted to take my biggest risk yet and join the school as a boarder in September. I was desperate to make a big change to my life and get things moving, and I couldn't see a better chance to do this than at the new school. It would be a new environment and a fresh routine. I loved my home but I was finding it too much of a challenge to move on in a place where my routines had been incorporated into every aspect of that life. To my surprise Mum and Ian encouraged this latest initiative and agreed to let me at least try boarding at the school; however, it was made very clear that I would continue to be weighed and if I wasn't managing we would go back to the original plan of being a day-girl. Gina was equally supportive; it was the first time she had seen me really excited and feeling positive about taking some risks.

Finally, the first induction day arrived. That morning I weighed my breakfast with the same accuracy as I had done since I left hospital, knowing full well that this time tomorrow the bowl of cereal in front of me wasn't going to be weighed. Driving away from the house made me realise just how much I was going to miss Mum and the happy, sheltered life we shared together. My time in the hospital and the months learning how to overcome my problems at home had brought us incredibly close; if it had not been for her endless patience, I knew I would never have had a chance of surviving outside hospital. Being the youngest with older sisters who had already flown the nest, I felt a sense of duty to stay at home and keep Mum company, though I knew she had Ian and also her friends. Mum assured me that she wasn't going to get lonely and that she had a number of ongoing tasks to keep her busy – nevertheless, I still hated the thought of leaving her in our big empty house.

As we approached the school my excitement-versus-nervousness ratio stood at about 90 per cent excitement to 10 per cent nerves. Walking towards the reception area in the boarding house we passed a number of smiling faces and a number looking just as daunted as Mum and me. I wondered how many other people would be coming in as a stranger like me, not knowing anyone around them. The housemistress was as welcoming as always and handed us our itinerary for the day. Top of the list was lunch – nothing like getting your teeth stuck into a challenge early! In the school canteen I spotted the cook Mum and I had met before to discuss the menu; she smiled and slipped off. When I came to the front of the line I looked disappointedly at the spread of potato salad, cooked meats, Scotch eggs, sausage rolls and cheeses – but from nowhere I was discreetly handed a plate with a plain chicken breast and baked potato. Mum and I both breathed a sigh of relief. I quickly added a few lettuce leaves and tomatoes to make my rather anaemic-looking plate of food less obvious, and we headed towards one of the empty tables.

This was going to be the first time in over a year that I was going to eat a meal that hadn't been weighed and scrutinised to within one calorie of accuracy. We were soon joined by another family and some students from the year above; with the distraction of talking and the awareness of how important it was to not make a fuss about what I was eating and draw attention to myself, I started my meal. Fifteen or so minutes later I put down my knife and fork but Mum looked at the remaining half a baked potato and gave me the look that conveyed, 'It needs to be more than that.' With a deep breath and a glance around me I picked up my knife and fork again.

Soon people were already lining up to try the various puddings also on offer: strawberries and cream, chocolate mousse, Pavlovas and fruit tarts – again, not my cup of tea. The students from the year above, on their best behaviour, took our plates and said that they would save me a place in the queue. Unsure what to do next, I followed behind nervously. Again the server recognised me and dished out a bowl of strawberries minus the cream. I knew the time ahead was going to be tough but I also knew there was a team behind the scenes looking out for me. As I left the dining hall I found the cook and thanked her for her thoughtful efforts.

The induction days were just as much fun as I hoped they would be, and saying goodbye to Mum wasn't the emotional separation that I was dreading. She looked thrilled to see me chatting away with the other students, and the organisation of the kitchen staff reassured her that I was in safe hands.

That night, as I climbed into my new bed, I felt happier than I had thought was possible. I could hear girls giggling in the bathroom and music playing in the next-door room and I still had the excitement of a school day ahead of me with more new people to meet.

The next morning I followed the group of girls into the dining hall for breakfast. I decided that Weetabix was a safe option, as I knew how many calories one Weetabix contains from my time in the unit, and there was no need to use the scales to measure a portion. Then came the milk. By this time I had struck up a friendship with a couple of girls who had been at the school since they were young, so I trusted they would know whether the milk was semi-skimmed or full fat. Luckily it was the former. The next step was pouring the 'right amount' onto my Weetabix. I watched the girls around me to get some indication of what was a normal portion. I tried hard to follow their example but after finishing my first Weetabix my bowl was dry, whereas theirs were still half-full of milk – clearly I had underdone this one.

Next up: the bread side of things. I opted for a brown roll rather than the two pieces of toast, as I thought it would look less obvious having no butter or jam on the roll than crunching through the dry toast. I tucked a pear into my pocket on the way out and I knew I still had a cereal bar and juice to get through in my room. I was worried that one of the other girls would come in and find me eating more and think I was really greedy. I felt bad enough thinking I was greedy myself, but I tried to rationalise that I probably wasn't eating any more than the rest of them and convinced myself that my cereal bar and fruit didn't contain too many calories more than they had consumed in the butter and jam on their toast.

Lunch the next day didn't run quite as smoothly as it had the previous day. With fewer parents and other visitors to talk to, more of the people around me noticed that my plate of food was different from theirs. I knew eventually someone would notice and had prepared myself for questions. I had two answers ready: the first that I used to be lactose intolerant when I was little – this got the butter, cream and cheese out of the picture – and the second that I had a very 'sensitive stomach', which meant that it was better for me to eat plainer meals – goodbye thick sauces and rich foods. To be honest, it was incredibly lucky that Food and Nutrition wasn't one of the A-level subjects the school offered, for despite being supposedly lactose intolerant I still ate yogurts and had milk on my cereal. Nobody said anything. I didn't know whether I had fobbed them off successfully or whether they saw straight through me but were too embarrassed to say anything.

I called Mum every day to tell her what my days were like, about the people I had met and how I was managing without my scales and the different food. I was loving every minute at the school. By the time Saturday arrived and Mum came to pick me up I was shattered but looking forward to another week. Walking towards the car with my bags I was hit by a pang of nerves: what if Mum thought I looked as if I had gained weight while I had been away? I didn't want her to think that weight was the only thing I had been thinking about, so I made a conscious effort not to jump right in and ask if she could see any changes in me, even though I was desperate to find out. Finally I couldn't avoid the subject of food and what it was like to be without my scales any longer. Mum was thrilled that I had survived a week of being independent but she looked nervously across at me as she said that I was looking tired and she was worried that I had cut myself short of food. I told her that I didn't think she had anything to worry about because I had that familiar feeling of discomfort. I was pinching my tummy and arms to see if they looked as big as they felt and was sure I had gained weight over the week. We would have to wait until Tuesday to see who was right.

Being at home I realised how exhausting it had been pretending to everyone around me that my problems with food were physiological rather than psychological. It was a relief seeing my normal yogurts in the fridge and my usual bread used to make my sandwiches, but I found the task of not weighing my food so much more difficult at home. At mealtimes Mum let me dish out what I thought was the right amount first, then she'd intervene, saying that I was a long way short of what I should be having. We were back to arguing over the correct-sized portion for a meal just as we had been all that time before I started seeing professionals. Whereas life with the scales had made meals less of an event, life without the scales made mealtimes incredibly long and tense. My poor estimation of what was the right portion size was clearly causing Mum's confidence in me to waver. Although she was pleased to see me excited about another week and pursuing the challenge of managing my diet myself, she reminded me that to keep enjoying it all I needed to up my intake.

By now my sessions with Gina had been reduced to one every two weeks, but we decided that it was still essential to be weighed weekly to address any fluctuations and to stop me from getting worked up with the worry that I was consistently gaining weight, so we arranged for me to be weighed weekly at the school medical centre.

To allay any of my fears that the school's scales might differ from the unit's we bought a new digital pair and calibrated them against my weight on the old pair. That first evening I had some bad news: I had been away only one week but I had already lost nearly a month of hard work and effort getting back within my target range. I dreaded telling Mum because I knew she'd be terrified. As my weight continued to drop over the following weeks Gina and Mum told me firmly that I was no longer allowed to participate in sporting activities until my weight started to increase and, if it did not, boarding would also stop. I felt so frustrated because I knew they were right and I could see exactly where I was going wrong, but even though I wanted to stop the weight loss and get back on track, when it came to the crunch I just couldn't do it.

The next week at school I did manage to make some changes to what I was eating. Mum had also helped me to find a new supply of higher-calorie cereal bars and juice drinks that I could keep in my room, and in that week my weight had improved. I had bought myself a little time to prove to everyone around me that I really did want to be more responsible. I was now allowed to take part in games lessons again but not in sport after school.

As time passed I became more experienced in how to stabilise my weight. I found a 'meal plan' that seemed to work and had a store of additional extras I could substitute if I was losing weight. I loved boarding so much that it was enough to motivate me, and I had made friends with a circle of girls who were great fun and bursting with confidence.

One lunchtime I noticed a girl I had never seen before who was painfully thin. Her clothes were hanging off her and I knew from the sunken look of her eyes that all was not well. I watched avidly as she got to the front of the lunch queue. Her friends were looking nervous as she walked away with a small pile of lettuce leaves. As I looked down at the sandwich, yogurt and fruit in front of me I felt incredibly ashamed and wondered what she thought when she looked at me.

Soon after, the girl disappeared from the scene. From the grapevine I learnt that she had been admitted into hospital. Her absence reminded me of where I had come from and gave me another flurry of determination that never again was I going to be 'the girl with anorexia'. I wasn't denying to myself that I still had a problem, but I didn't want to lose the control I had that enabled me to cope on my own without everyone around me needing to know. But the questions that had arisen in me when I first saw her made me feel even more conscious about my body image. Despite my determination to keep going, the battle on the inside continued to require constant attention.

As the terms went by my weight mainly remained stable and for once I didn't have the ongoing nightmare of always having to gain weight. During my sessions with Gina we faced the new challenges that arose along with becoming more independent: spending nights at friends' houses and managing breakfast in the morning, going out for meals without Mum to guide me, and even facing my concerns about how many calories are in a glass of wine! I asked Gina and Mum to make sure that from now on only those on a 'need to know' basis would know what I weighed and how my appointment with the scales went each week. Basically, that included Mum, Gina, the consultant and Pam, the nurse who weighed me at school – I didn't want Ian, Beth or Jenny to know. Ultimately, I didn't want people to look at me in terms of weight any more.

After about a year of being at my new school I was thrilled that one of the boys in my year had started to phone in the evening and meet up with my friends and me when we were out at weekends. A few weeks later I introduced Mum and Ian to Tom, my first boyfriend. I didn't tell him anything about my illness.

The idea of bringing Tom home to supper was a total nightmare, as I still wasn't yet eating the same meals as the rest of my family and I rarely ever sat down to eat with them. Usually I would eat earlier and come to chat with them at the table. Mum and I talked the evening over beforehand: how we were going to make things look normal, what meal we could have to make it as easy as possible and what time we would eat. It turned out to be fun and soon we became pretty apt at producing these 'relaxed' family meals. I never looked too far into the future, as I did not want to worry about the problem of telling Tom the truth.

A few months down the line Tom and I had become very close. We were spending a lot of time together and I started to ask Mum whether she thought I should let him in on my secret about my past (I had told only one of my very close friends at school during a difficult patch). In the end one of my close family friends beat me to it and inadvertently let it out of the bag. She was waitressing with Tom and had assumed that after so long together he must have known, so she asked him how I was getting on. Later that night I got a rather confused phone call from Tom asking if it was true that two years earlier I had been admitted into hospital with anorexia. I finally let my barriers down and told him about what had happened and how it still affected my life. After having to tell him unexpectedly I felt a huge sense of relief, as though a burden had been lifted off my shoulders. The next day when I saw him I reiterated that I didn't want anything to change – he didn't need to 'look after me' or worry about me in that sense. Tom wholly understood and I felt so much more relaxed not having to worry whether he would notice that I didn't have gravy on my chicken or that I had yogurt and not ice cream. When I returned to school after my meeting with Gina he always met me to check everything had gone all right and that I was OK.

As time went on my periods returned and I was more independent about managing and preparing my meals. When I next met my consultant I hoped that my growing happiness and freedom would show him how grateful we all were for everything he had done and give him a sense of hope in a world where frequent readmission and relapse can make you wonder where the struggle ever ends. In spite of my misgivings that without my medication I would begin to deteriorate, I trusted his judgement and reassurance that I was no longer relying on the medication to the extent that I was when it was first prescribed. He set out a time schedule to reduce it very gradually, and coming off my medication meant that I no longer felt under the stigma of being 'crazy'. I now felt more in control of my thoughts and less as though my brain was a separate entity punishing my body.

As I approached the midway mark of my final year at school my 14-month relationship with Tom came to an end as we seemed to have grown apart, and I'll be the first to admit that I wasn't the world's easiest girlfriend; at times I felt totally consumed by my eating disorder and so wrought with anxiety that I couldn't concentrate on what was happening around me.

I began to face the future. I started looking at the different university prospectuses and thinking seriously about my ambition to study medicine, though I knew my determination to enter such a competitive environment made Mum very anxious. Throughout my time in hospital I had always let it be known how much I wanted to study medicine, yet I was afraid that my complicated medical record would damage my chances. Despite her fears that I was taking on more than I could handle, Mum never tried to persuade me to redirect my excitement about studying medicine towards another career path – yet again, she was behind me all the way.

CHAPTER 5

Living with Alice

It feels like years have passed between then and now. Although I still haven't found a totally effective cure for my eating disorder, I have become more independent than I ever thought would be possible. After months of writing and rewriting application forms, personal statements and interviews I have finally accepted an offer to study medicine at university. I know that should I slip up or lose control and find myself back at the GP's door I will not only jeopardise my sought-after place at university but ultimately I will minimise the chances of any future in a medical career. On some levels I think I was at least fortunate to have developed the problem when I was still young, as I had the opportunity to establish a method of coping and the chance to have a few years of stability behind me before trying to prove my staying power.

Leaving my school was heartbreaking. I didn't want to leave my tight network of friends, the vibrant atmosphere and the security of a routine. My friends did come to learn about my problems. Some of the girls I opened up to, a few asked out of concern when they could see me struggling, and I suppose a few just guessed. They all respected that weight was a sensitive issue to me, and restricted their talk about dieting to when I wasn't around. When we went out for girlie meals they were fantastic at thinking ahead and booking restaurants where they knew I would feel comfortable, and nothing was ever said about my reluctance to experiment with different foods. After two years of living together I knew their absence, when I was back at home, would leave an enormous gap.

As I approached my eighteenth birthday I was aware that eventually my time under the watchful eye of my consultant and his team of miracle workers would have to come to an end. I was now becoming more willing to deal with my tendency to misinterpret compliments about 'keeping well' so that I no longer had to unload them onto Gina during my next appointment. I felt ready to move on again. But I could sense how nervous Mum was about losing the support of the unit; I knew she felt I was still incredibly fragile and that should things start to go wrong without the attention of the professionals I would very quickly be back to the point we had found ourselves at three years before.

My final appointment with my consultant was probably the strangest yet. Since that first assessment meeting I had felt such a range of attitudes towards him. I had hated him for his invasive, blunt analysis of my health and our family situation; I had felt frustration and fear at his ability always to read between the lines and see the truth when I was trying my hardest to keep it from him, bitterness at being 'punished' and put on to bed-rest, but, most overwhelmingly, gratitude. I'll never forget the look on his face during that final meeting: he looked proud and satisfied. Thanks to his own and his team's adaptability and consistency, I was being signed off as a happy, independent and positive patient rather than one whose record was probably safest kept at the top of the pile just in case.

I can't avoid admitting the pressure I put on those I'm closest to for 'honest opinions' about my weight and appearance. When Mum voices her concerns that I'm looking tired and thin I become defensive and frustrated, saying that I wish everyone wasn't always on my case. However, should she ever say that she thinks I'm doing well, I jump to the conclusion that she thinks I'm gaining weight and then I become incredibly agitated and uptight to the point where I usually start making those wrongly calculated cuts to my diet. I hope that in the future I'll become more confident about my body perception and less reliant on what those around me see when they look at me.

It infuriates me when people talk about 'choosing' to become an anorexic; I don't remember making that choice and I can't flick the 'off' button just as easily. Seeing it written down I can convince myself that I am going to strive for a full recovery, I will put the right amount of milk on my cereal this week, but in practice it doesn't run that smoothly. Something tells me that skipping it just once won't matter and then as soon as I've thought about it and am making the conscious 'choice' to eat more than I could get away with I feel greedy. I even begin to worry that perhaps I was destined to be obese but by having an eating disorder I stopped it and that if I let go now I'm going to be a hundred times larger than I am now. 'Complicated' doesn't begin to describe it.

After I have slowly become less of a responsibility and a drain on Mum's time, thoughts and efforts, I think Jenny has started to accept that I never intended any of this to happen and that it wasn't a ploy for attention. Watching me trying to adapt around my fears and compulsions about food, Jenny has become less abrasive and more understanding about the things I've missed out on and the limitations I still experience in everyday life. Whenever I start to lose the battle of control and make mistakes, Jenny is my first port of call. She is one of the very few who can get through to me when I'm swamped in my thoughts and give me the reality in black and white; with Jenny there's no sidestepping the issue when things go wrong. Beth, in contrast, tends to lie low during my mealtimes and rarely confronts me on the ongoing trials of my eating disorder. In the past we've realised that we don't work overly well together trying to combat my eating problems, and although I know she's always there ready and waiting to help, we tend to avoid discussing the issue whenever possible.

Although my relationship with Nuala and my other old friends was a little restrained while I was away at boarding school, now that I spend more time at home during my gap year before going to medical school and I see Nuala more regularly we're back to the sister-like bond that we shared for so long. While I was unwell we shared experiences that two friends should never have to encounter, but for some reason we did and there's no one I would rather have had beside me through it all than her. I am confident that we will always play a part in each other's life no matter what's thrown at us next.

I hope that those who know me would agree that I haven't lost my positive attitude or my zeal for having fun, but that I have become a little more realistic in understanding that you can't predict everything. Sadly, Dad hasn't been close enough to watch these changes taking place. I can remember years ago Beth and Jenny encouraging Dad to take more of an active part in my growing up, I was still young enough for him to learn more about me and the person I was. I know my eating disorder made this more complicated and made me harder to approach. However, I can also say that if things could be done again differently I think he probably would have become more involved in the hope that when I re-emerged into the outside world there wouldn't be the gap between us that there is today. It's difficult arranging visits to spend time with him because I know he'll find my behaviour towards food confusingly irrational and totally alien to the plucky Alice of five years ago. Beth and Jenny are ready and waiting for when I take this next risk and start making bridges to bring him more up to date on the person I am today.

I find it so difficult to tie up all the loose ends that still remain after writing 'my story'. Not only is it incredibly exhausting and emotionally draining to look back over four such life-changing years, but many of those loose ends are what I'm still living with today. Foodwise, I don't have a meal plan written down in black and white but I do have a mental list of what I need to eat in a day. Even though I sometimes experiment with slight variations, I do, by and large, eat exactly the same day in and day out, with the exception of different suppers (which are all planned and portioned out to meet the 'normal' supper calorie requirement). It doesn't frustrate me or hold me back from doing the things I want to do; if I want to go out with my friends, I'll buy a sandwich before we go, eat supper earlier or take something with me in case there's nothing suitable where we're going. Sometimes I do get out the kitchen scales when I'm feeling unsure of how much is the right amount. I'm still taking risks, but they're carefully controlled not only to reduce my anxiety but also to prevent me from relying on my poor judgement of how much I need to eat.

Every week Mum and I have our own private appointment with the bathroom scales. I still haven't quite mastered the blissful stability that I managed to secure while I was at school. There seems to be a pattern of me getting to within my target range, freaking myself out, making underhand cutbacks during the following week, getting back on the scales a week later and finding that I've cut out too much and having to increase my calorie intake. On reflection I can so easily see the mistakes I'm making and the additional stress I continue to create for myself. However, somewhere throughout the course of a week this sense of logic tends to wander, and if I know that last week I gained weight, no matter how determined I am to maintain that week's efforts, when it comes to the crunch, the mental agony that accompanies eating what I know is the minimum anyway is easily relieved by 'opting out', backing away from the confrontation and having the lower-calorie option.

The fear of gaining more weight than I 'need to' can still influence and sometimes override the positive, rational thoughts inside me. Sometimes, especially when I'm tired or grumpy, I get so fed up with having to wait for my anxiety to go down that I think 'Stuff it!' and I cheat. I hope that eventually some day eating will become a less 'conscious' activity and I'll learn to be able to eat everything I need to keep my body healthy without the mental argument that goes on in my head.

However, I haven't lost my nerve or given up. Every day I'm gaining in confidence and with more experience of what life can offer if I push myself to be a part of it I'm learning that I want to take more from it. One of my proudest achievements after leaving school is travelling around Croatia, Greece and Turkey with my great friend Kirsty. I didn't want Kirsty to see me as an added responsibility, but I needed to tell her of the bugs that were still in my system and ask her to keep an eye on me. There were testing times; the agitation I experienced being on a ferry for over 24 hours and not having anywhere to relieve my anxiety about not doing any exercise, the hassle of finding a sandwich bar that would make me up a sandwich with just salad – no butter, mayo or cheese – the nights of being lost (with our 15kg backpacks) in the rain at ten o'clock knowing that I still had to eat supper. But the majority of the time was spent thinking just how amazing it all was. We met some great people, dived off outstandingly beautiful rocky coasts into perfectly crystalline seas and collapsed in fits of giggles at our lame attempts at erecting the tent!

As I landed at the airport I was bursting with excitement, to have a long-needed hug from Mum at last, but also nervous about how I was going to convince her that I hadn't intended to lose weight while away – it's just that travelling around had taken its toll. I told Mum that I intended to get back within my target weight range as soon as possible. Coming home with so many fantastic stories made me feel so much more independent and liberated from the limitations of my eating disorder.

The reality that I still have medical school ahead of me to prove to myself and everyone around me that I'm not going to be held back by this illness any more is incredibly exciting. I try not to think about how I'm going to manage the food there or whether I'll need to make up any more cunning excuses. I know it's impractical, but the dream is too perfect to puncture with the reality that not everything will be plain sailing and that considerations will eventually have to be made if I'm going to make it through.

Up to this day I have no idea how I climbed out of my misery, how it was that I managed to control my exercise and finally take responsibility for everything that I was doing to avoid getting better. I think it was probably a combination of a number of pivotal moments: reaching the all-time low on bed-rest, feeling 'left behind' and isolated by my patient peer group, being awarded the bonus of walks in return for my efforts dedicated to recovery, being given a 'clean slate' and a change of environment, spending more time with my friends and seeing the happiness in Mum's face as she watches me laugh and enjoy life.

My greatest advantage throughout this entire journey has been the relationship I share with Mum. Even at the hardest of times she never gave up or lost hope that there was something that could be done to help me to find the old values that I used to live my life by: family, friends and fun. Today I'm able to be the positive person I am only because Mum taught me to see the future as a door of opportunities rather than a threat of disasters. During my time in hospital the staff often recognised the close bond that we shared and would remind me how lucky I was to have someone so selfless and committed by my side. Our friendship has been at the heart of my recovery. Even at my most lonely times when I felt that no one understood me, I knew she was always thinking about me and waiting for the moment when I would give her the signal that I was finally ready to accept that I was being beaten by an illness and needed help. How can you ever really thank someone for being your everything? I hope that one day I find the answer and can prove to her that despite her lack of confidence she did an amazing job.

This might not be the 'done and dusted' ending to my eating disorder that we're all hoping for one day soon, but if I remember back to how dire our situation was, things are looking pretty good. I am in control of my eating disorder and with the help of my family, friends and the professionals I no longer feel trapped or isolated in a world of anxiety. Writing this account has been an incredibly purging process for me; as the pages have turned I've subconsciously started to accept responsibility for more of what has happened. I don't think I could ever have prevented developing the eating disorder but I do think I ran away from it for too long. I convinced myself that I didn't have a problem for a long time after my diagnosis was confirmed by experienced professionals. I kept telling myself that I wasn't thin enough to have anorexia or that I was eating too much.

To a large extent I still find myself falling into the same trap today. I will avoid confronting the fact that it happened and that I did have a serious problem, which I couldn't solve myself. I still haven't put my various excuses about not wanting salad dressing or avoiding dairy products totally to bed. It's a combination of shame about losing personal control of something so natural and instinctive as eating and also anxiety about defying people's expectations about how an anorexic should behave; I'm concerned that people will think I'm the stereotypical teenager, pretending for the sake of attracting attention. I wish I could reveal the secret of my recovery and bring hope to all those people fighting the battle against an eating disorder. I don't really know how it happened, but I managed to confront my fears and take the risk of finding something more important to me than my weight.

Resources

Books

Clare Beeken and Rosanna Greenstreet, *My Body My Enemy: My Thirteen-year Battle with Anorexia Nervosa*, Thorsons, 1997

Rachel Bryant-Waugh and Bryan Lask, *Eating Disorders: A Parents' Guide*, Brunner-Routledge, 2004

Kate Chisholm, *Hungry Hell: What it's Really like to be Anorexic*, Short Books, 2002

Dee Dawson, *Anorexia and Bulimia: A Parents' Guide to Recognising Eating Disorders and Taking Control*, Vermilion, 2001

EDA Carer's Guide, Eating Disorders Association, 2002

Christopher Freeman, *Overcoming Anorexia Nervosa, A Self-help Guide Using Cognitive Behavioral Techniques*, Constable & Robinson Ltd, 2002

Grainne Smith, *Anorexia and Bulimia in the Family*, John Wiley & Sons, 2004

Janet Treasure, *Anorexia Nervosa: A Survival Guide for Families, Friends and Sufferers*, Psychology Press, 1997, repr. Brunner-Routledge, 2003

Useful contacts
The Eating Disorders Association
First Floor, Wensum House
103 Prince of Wales Road
Norwich
NR1 1DW
Tel: 01603 619090
Website: www.edauk.com

Something Fishy
Dedicated to raising awareness and providing support to people with eating disorders.
Website: www.somethingfishy.org

PIATKUS BOOKS

If you have enjoyed reading this book, you may be interested in other titles published by Piatkus. These include:

All Piatkus titles are available from:

Piatkus Books , c/o Bookpost , PO Box 29, Douglas, Isle Of Man,
IM99 1BQ

Telephone (+44) 01624 677237
Fax (+44) 01624 670923
Email; bookshop@enterprise.net
Free Postage and Packing in the United Kingdom
Credit Cards accepted. All Cheques payable to Bookpost

Prices and availability subject to change without prior notice. Allow 14
days for delivery. When placing orders please state if you do not wish to
receive any additional information.